Self Treatment for over 60 common
ailments and conditions.

Do-It-Yourself Natural Health:
Natural Health Trio

Acupressure, Aromatherapy
& Herbal Therapy

John Sherman, Ph.D, OTR, CST

Publishers Advocate Award Winner

New Found Therapies Publications
Monterey, California

Do-It-Yourself Natural Health: Natural Health Trio.
by John Sherman, Ph.D, OTR, CST
ISBN# 0970941129

Other books by the author:

Do-It-Yourself Natural Health Pocket Reference.
by John Sherman, Ph.D, OTR, CST
ISBN# 0970941137

Do-It-Yourself Natural Health
by John Sherman, MS, OTR, CST
ISBN# 0970941110

Under Pressure
by John Sherman, MS, OTR, CST
ISBN# 0970941102

Fast and Easy Pressure Point Relief
by John Sherman, MS, OTR, CST
ISBN# 1877809837

Fast and Easy Pressure Point Relief Companion Book
by John Sherman, MS, OTR, CST
ISBN# 1877809845

IMPORTANT - PLEASE READ!

Cover design: George Foster
info@fostercovers.com

About the author:

Dr. John Sherman has been a practicing Licensed Occupational Therapist and Certified Shiatsu Therapist for over thirty-three years. He is a former Instructor and Assistant Professor of physical disabilities at Texas Woman's University and San Jose State University. Born and raised in Boston, he now resides with his wife, Dr. Diane Sherman, in Monterey, California.

Dedication:

To Hanna, Kristin, Lauren, Sarah, and Wyatt.

Table of Contents

Table of Contents

Table of Contents

Table of Contents

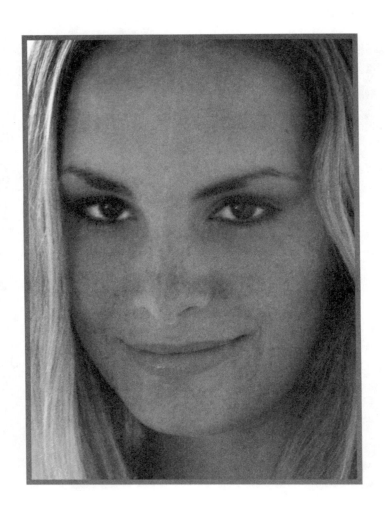

Foreword

This book, an introduction to acupressure, aromatherapy and herbal therapy, contains the basic information for natural health relief. Acupressure facilitates the alleviation or lessening of pain and discomfort by activating specific areas of the body, literally creating neuromuscular and circulatory changes, through massage and pressure. Aromatherapy positively affects the limbic system of the brain. It provides a calming setting for natural treatments and increases the effectiveness of natural therapies. Herbal therapy is the natural approach to healing by treating the entire body. Herbs have a long history of healing and maintaining health and wellness

This is not a book that should sit on your shelf. Keep it in your car's glove compartment, by your television, or under your pillow so you will have instant access to this healing information.

You will learn the fundamentals about acupressure, herbs, and aromatherapy, but the real benefits come from the natural approach to good health. Implementing natural therapies that have minimal side effects is a sensible, healthy approach to wellness. Natural therapies empower everyone to choose from many therapies to customize a lifestyle of natural health and wellness.

Introduction

In the summer of 2000, George W. Bush, then a candidate for the Presidency of the United States, addressing a rally of supporters, stated that "the United States has the best healthcare system in the world." Also in 2000, JAMA, the official journal of the American Medical Association, published the results of a survey of healthcare services in thirteen countries around the world (July 26, 2000-284.483.485). The survey focused on sixteen health indicators that were considered factors in measuring healthcare quality, and ranked the countries according to the results. The rankings of the countries were as follows:

> Japan, Sweden, Canada, France, Australia, Spain, Finland, the Netherlands, the United Kingdom, Denmark, Belgium, the United States, and Germany.

The United States ranked no better than twelfth.

This poor performance was confirmed by the World Health Organization, using different indicators, ranked the United States as15th among 25 industrialized countries, primarily because the U.S has not developed a strong primary care system available to all who needed medical care.

Introduction

The results of international surveys document the high availability of technology in the United States. In another WHO survey, among 29 countries, the United States is second only to Japan in the availability of magnetic resonance imaging units and computed tomography scanners per million population. However, Japan ranks highest for providing the best primary care services, according to the healthcare survey, whereas the United States ranks among the lowest.

The JAMA article also suggests that states with wide divisions of wealth appear to have lower levels of primary care services and availability of technology for the poor. The JAMA article also sites 225,000 deaths per year that were related to the following factors:

12,000 deaths/year from unnecessary surgery.

7,000 deaths/year from medication errors in hospitals.

20,000 deaths/year from other errors in hospitals.

80,000 deaths/year from nosocomial infections in hospitals.

106,000 deaths/year from nonerror, adverse effects of medications.

Introduction

Errors in medication and hospital-related incidences ranks third in causes of death in the U.S. behind heart disease and cancer. Estimates for causes of death in 2005 by the American Heart Association from heart disease are 920,000 and by the American Cancer Society from major forms of cancer are 430,000.

Most of us in the U.S. have relied on governmental agencies, such as the Food and Drug Administration, to oversee the research, development, trial studies, manufacturing, and distributing of medications. We have grown to rely upon the FDA's judgment of approving prescription medications that are *safe and effective,* because the FDA has stated that this is one of their primary functions and obligations to the public. The key words are *safe and effective.* Because the FDA has been empowered to insure that medications available to the public have been impartially evaluated and approved, we have accepted their findings and recommendations as impartial and objective.

Today we are seeing evidence that standards are not necessarily applied in a uniform procedure. For example, the FDA received numerous complaints from the public and healthcare professionals about

Introduction

safety and side effects of medications with cox2 inhibitors. These complaints related to stomach and intestinal bleeding, stroke, and cardiovascular risks. Two years of complaints passed before the FDA, under intense pressure, ordered manufacturers remove the cox2 inhibitors from pharmacy shelves. With some suspected arm-twisting the FDA, by a boardroom approval of one vote, decided that these medications could be placed back on the pharmacy shelves for distribution by prescription with a warning label stating the possible serious cardiovascular effects. Shortly after that decision, the medications were again pulled from the shelves.

If governmental agencies are vulnerable to external pressures, our trust and best interests about our health and welfare are being compromised. To protect our safety and health, we have trusted these governmental agencies to watch out for our welfare, but we have learned over the past several years that these same agencies do not act in our best interests.

Developing a new medication is a risky business. The cost for researching and developing a new medication is about 100 million dollars. About three dozen new medications are submitted each year to the

Introduction

Food and Drug Administration for approval. Only a few of these submitted drugs are considered "breakthrough" medications. The remaining are considered "copy cat" drugs, similar to ones already available by prescription. Any large corporation is aware that investors, stockholders and other parties closely monitor the costs of producing new medications and expect a positive return on their investment. Marketing, distributing, and branding a new medication are part of business expenses, and the budget for promoting a new medication may be as much or more than the research and development costs. Corporations are also keenly aware of the time factor for exclusive rights to a new medication.

We are a nation of medication consumers. Nearly 50% of all people in the United States are taking one prescription medication, and half of them are taking three or more prescription medications. This does not included the hundreds of thousands of over-the-counter medications sold every year.

Through the power of marketing and promoting, advertisers are convincing us that we need their particular medication, prescription or over-the-counter drug, to live better, love better, and feel better. By purposeful design we are slowly conditioned that taking prescription and over-the-counter

Introduction

drugs is our best and only avenue to good health. Our developed frame of reference is that we have choices of several medications for a specific condition. Actually a few pharmaceutical companies are promoting their own medication, suggesting their product is superior, even though the medications are similar. This is called *product differentiation.*

Healthcare is a profit-motivated industry. The 2003 Money Magazine article on prescription medications revealed that for every dollar pharmaceutical companies invested in advertising and marketing, the company realized four dollars in sales. Traditionally, pharmaceutical companies have marketed exclusively to physicians. This was profitable, but they realized an untapped market of consumers existed. Recent promotions have been directed to the consumers, encouraging them to talk with their doctor or healthcare professionals to see if a specific medication was right for them. Consumers were probably not adequately knowledgeable to understand the potential side effects of this medication, but they clearly grasped the message that this medication could be the right one for them. They understood the prompt to talk with their doctor. Consumers took the bait, visited their doctor, and sales soared.

Introduction

Dr. Simon Markind, M.D. a physiatrist at the Auburn Health and Rehabilitation Center, stated that medications have two negative effects for one positive effect. This generalization was a caution to other physicians and healthcare professionals of side effects when using a medication or combination of medications. Unless a reference source, such as the *Physician's Desk Reference*, was available these side effects were not common knowledge.

Today, because of laws on consumer information, companies are required to report side effects of medications as part of public awareness. Most companies comply with these requirements, but the Money Magazine article asserts that about 25% of pharmaceutical companies omitted mentioning significant side effects. In addition, some ads mentioned side effects while focusing on a pleasing image. Another technique was listing the side effects interrupting the list with a positive interjection or testimonial. The human brain tends to focus on a pleasing visual image rather than a verbal listing of side effects, and it tends to retain the last part of the message. These subtle and effective techniques have been proven to sway prospective customers to retain the positive message and suppress the negative information.

Introduction

Pharmaceutical companies realized that promoting to the general public has a powerful effect on sales. Moreover, advertisers promote products and services that depend on the consumer returning to purchase that product on a regular basis. Some will offer a free sample or trial period betting the consumer will keep and use the product on a regular basis. They may continue contacting the interested consumer for continuing the product or service with special offers or long-term commitment bargains. Very few advertisers promote products and services that are purchased once, because return business helps assure a stable flow of revenue. This is critical when developing a business plan that has a high degree of accuracy for projecting sales and revenue. In plain terms, the goal is to keep the customer coming back.

Millions of people are using prescribed medications for specific health reasons. These medications add quality to their lives. But there are also millions who believe that a particular medication might alleviate some mild maladies, so they visit a local pharmacy or make an appointment with their doctor. How did these people learn about these medications? They did not read medical journals or conduct research, many probably saw or heard of an ad in a magazine or

Introduction

television. We, the consumer, are consumed by marketing programs, advertisements, and promotions. If we are frustrated by rising medical costs, overwhelmed with medication expenses, and discouraged by the lack of progress reforming healthcare, maybe the answer we seek is outside our traditional healthcare system.

One approach for change is climbing out of the rut and taking charge of our own healthcare. We do not need to abandon our present healthcare system, but we have many alternative healthcare products and services that are proven to be extremely beneficial for general health and wellness. If we examine the list of the thirteen countries in the *JAMA* article, nearly everyone of them embrace forms of alternative healthcare as common practice in their countries.

In the last decade U.S. physicians are using alternative approaches for treating common ailments. Today about one-third of physicians incorporate forms of alternative healthcare into their patient treatments. About one-third acknowledge the value of alternative healthcare and recommend the use of some therapies. The remaining one-third are physicians opposed to alternative healthcare, stating more research is needed. In fact, alternative healthcare therapies have 3,000 years of proven effectiveness.

Introduction

If you are intrigued by alternative healthcare therapies, the first question might be who can benefit from these therapies? A classic response might be "everyone." If alternative healthcare was for everyone, all other forms of healthcare would be obsolete. However, if alternative healthcare was without substance, it would not have survived thousands of years. The evidence is that alternative healthcare has been around for many generations and is practiced by millions of people around the world every day.

Alternative healthcare has a very fundamental philosophy. Alternative health-care addresses a basic approach to the health of the human body, mind, and spirit. Alternative healthcare celebrates "wellness." Wellness includes the total person for health and   well-being through natural approaches, such as herbs, Yoga, pressure points, medita-tion, and much more. Maintaining a balance of a lifestyle can prevent many illnesses and maladies. One of the strongest points for alternative healthcare is minimal, if any, side effects. However, certain forms of alternative healthcare, such as acupuncture and herbal medicine, require the skills of a trained professional. Licensed acupuncturists and Oriental Medical Doctors are licensed professionals who can conduct effective treatments.

Introduction

Most alternative healthcare therapies do not require the level of professional credentials as an acupuncturist or Oriental Medical Doctor. In fact, many therapies can be conducted by anyone who invests a few hours of study. Through self-study, many can learn some of the basics of these therapies for effect self-treatment.

Here is an approach that may help you make that decision. If you take a serious look at your lifestyle, that is your daily routine, what you do, and how you do it, this will help pinpoint specific activities of your lifestyle. These are called *activities of daily living.*

Activities of daily living are basic activities of our lifestyle. If we are sometimes hampered by aches, pain, discomfort, fatigue, or stress, and if these conditions are a *mild* or *moderate* interference with daily activities, we can learn natural health treatments to alleviate many of these conditions.

Three more reasons make these therapies worth investigating: fast, safe, and inexpensive. Acupressure, Yoga, and massage can reduce dozens of conditions, such as aches, pain, anxiety, and fatigue. Because the treatments are natural, no medications are needed to reduce or eliminate these conditions. Benefits are felt almost immediately, instead of waiting up to

Introduction

an hour for the body to absorb a medication, and these therapies can stimulate circulation and rid the body of toxins in minutes.

Aromatherapy and meditation, can reduce stress, fatigue, and anxiety in just a few minutes. These therapies positively affect the limbic system, including the pituitary gland and hypothalamus, that regulate the autonomic nervous system for heart rate, body temperature, and food and water intake. Inhaling eucalyptus can help breathing and reduce feelings of stuffiness. Inhaling lavender can provide a calming effect and reduce tension and stress.

Ingesting common herbs can provide fast relief for conditions and have long-term positive effects on the body. For example, the herbs of parsley and peppermint help to rid bad breath and aid digestion. An 8 oz. cup of ginger tea can quickly help rid nausea, indigestion, and cramps. Kava, St. John's Wort, Ginseng, and Saw Palmetto help to build and keep a healthy immune system. Research results from the American Botanical Council recently published the findings that St. John's Wort was more effective relieving depression than a commonly prescription drug (May, 2005).

Even the person who believes his or her health level is fine can benefit from natural

Introduction

therapies. Using natural healthcare therapies in place of prescription and over-the-counter medications will reduce the risk of long-term side effects associated with some of them.

In my article that appeared in BottomLine/Health newsletter (July, 2004), I described a sensible approach to treat common ailments and conditions using acupressure, herbal therapy, and aromatherapy. Of the available natural healthcare therapies I selected these three for effective self-help treatment. In my professional experience, acupressure addresses the immediate need for relief from conditions and ailments, aromatherapy helps the mind and body to relax and facilitates treatments, and herbs provide properties for long-term health and wellness.

For example, HEADACHES on pages 120 and 121 illustrates *seven pressure points* for relief, *orange blossom* for aromatherapy, and *cayenne, chamomile,* and *lavender* for helpful herbs. Pressure points are listed from head to toe for easy reference, and there is no particular order for activating them. Deciding which pressure points are most effective is very individual, so each person may find several of the seven that work best for them. Cayenne may be taken by capsule, but many people prefer to drink chamomile and lavender as a warm tea.

Introduction

INDIGESTION on pages 128 and 129 illustrates *four pressure points* for fast relief, *peppermint* for aromatherapy, and *Cat's claw, chamomile, comfrey, fennel seed, ginger, lemon balm, and peppermint* for helpful herbs. Note that the herbs are listed in alphabetical order. One client prefers peppermint tea to aid indigestion, and another person prefers eating a slice of ginger root for fast relief. Try different herbs for their effectiveness, but not at the same time.

A third condition is JET LAG on pages 132 and 133. This condition is a collection of symptoms causing discomfort and sluggishness. In addition to using pressure points, aromatherapy, and herbal therapy, additional treatments of *massage* and *physical activity* are indicated. Most of the pressure points are activated by pressing and massaging, but several points only require finger pressure, such Yin Tang, the point on the bridge of the nose. This point is also referred as The Third Eye. Pressure points close to the surface or over bony areas require mild to moderate pressure for activation. These points should not be massaged, because the delicate tissue under the point can easily damage. As a caution, these points will be indicated by the words PRESS ONLY next to the description.

Introduction

These three examples demonstrate the ease of learning and using acupressure, herbal therapy, and aromatherapy. The positive values associated with alternative healthcare therapies are intriguing.

One positive aspect of alternative healthcare therapies that has not been discussed is the cost. Learning and using acupressure for self-treatments has virtually no cost except for the resources for learning, such as an illustrated book or weekend class. Aromatherapy can be a few dollars for a candle to light or atomizer to spray the essence into the air. Nearly all the herbs in this book are standardized by manufacturing and available in tablets, capsules, tinctures, teas, creams, or raw form for less than $10.00.

A clear distinction between *herbal therapy* and *herbal medicine* is important. In this book, herbal therapy refers to common herbs found in the kitchen, garden, or readily available at many drug stores or health food stores. Examples of these common herbs are cinnamon, ginger, saw palmetto, St. John's wort, chamomile, and peppermint. Herbal medicine refers to a skilled level using herbs and herbal mixtures for treating chronic or serious conditions, and should be administered by a trained professional. If you

Introduction

are taking prescription medications or under a doctor's care for an ailment, inform your doctor if you are considering herbal treatments. If you have adverse effects from taking herbs, consult your doctor.

Healthcare professionals are available to assist with information and education, and the benefits from all natural healthcare are enormous. Before time and energy are distracted, take the small amount of effort to learn and benefit from these therapies.

You will notice that very few brand names are offered in this book. This is to allow every reader the choice to seek the resources that can provide the best products and services that suit them. Those that I offer are simply references of companies that I have found to be reliable for product and service quality. There is no remuneration, and I encourage each person to select companies and vendors of choice. You are welcome to contact me at my website with questions and comments at

www.diynaturalhealth.com.
or   **www.diynaturalhealth.net.**
or email at
        information@diynaturalhealth.com
I wish you good health and happiness.

John Sherman, Ph.D, OTR, CST.

Most Important:
Breathe

Breathing correctly is essential for increasing the flow of oxygen into our blood and helping us to relax. Without sufficient oxygen our system cannot function effectively. Learning how to properly breathe, even for a few seconds, can dramatically increase the oxygen exchange and reduce stress.

Place your hands on your abdomen, using your navel as a reference point, and breathe so that you are able to feel your abdomen expand and contract. Repeat this exercise several times using a slow, comfortable pace, and soon you will feel the tension leave your muscles and your mind clear. Correct breathing is the beginning of acupressure and aromatherapy therapies. The relaxed body and mind enhances the effectiveness of therapy treatments.

Taking a few seconds to correctly breathe can reduce stress, anxiety, muscle tension, and fatigue. Schedule times during the day to breathe for relaxation, perhaps several times in the morning and afternoon. Mark the times on a daily calendar or electronic reminder. Learning how to breathe properly is an essential first step to optimize alternative healthcare therapies.

Chi and Meridians.

Ancient philosophers and physicians believed that all of us have energy, or life force, that flows within us. The Chinese refer to this energy as Chi. Chi is directed through the body by specific paths or meridians. Along these meridians are points that control the flow of Chi. When Chi flows freely in body, we are in balance and in harmony with the world and the people around us. When these points or gates become blocked, not allowing Chi to flow, we experience disharmony through illness, discomfort and pain.

Chi is composed of two elements, Yin and Yang. Yin is the feminine element and Yang is the masculine element. The contrast between the two is stark, usually represented by black and white, but also represented as light and dark, right and left, good and evil, or any opposing forces that give us balance and purpose to life.

Yin and Yang are not static but dynamic. These two change just as winter changes into spring and then to summer, or just as night gives way to the rising sun, to daylight, then to sunset, and to dusk. Because they are constantly changing, balance of the two is necessary for harmony.

Chi and Meridians.

In order to bring Chi into balance and create harmony in our lives, we can use various exercises and techniques, such as meditation, coordination activities, and abdominal breathing.

One fundamental belief about imbalance is that the flow of Chi in the body has been blocked, thus preventing the life force from flowing freely through us. One way to open the pathways of the Chi is to open the gates of its passage -- our pressure points.

We instinctively use pressure points without realizing it. If we have a headache, we rub our head. If we have an aching neck, we rub it. If our eyes are tired and sore, we rub them. By doing so, we are in fact reopening those gates or pressure points that allow healing to take place. We are subconsciously finding our own pressure points and releasing the Chi that has been trapped, allowing it to flow throughout the body.

Chi and Meridians

The meridians are the specific paths through which Chi, or life energy, flows in our body. Some of the pathways are for Yin, some, for Yang. There are twelve pairs of meridians located on the extremities and two vessels, meridians not in pairs, located on the midline of the body. Each of the meridians has a mirror on the opposite side of the body.

The Six Meridians Located in the Legs

B	Urinary Bladder—Yang
Kd	Kidney—Yin
Lv	Liver—Yin
St	Stomach—Yang
Sp	Spleen and Pancreas—Yin
Gb	Gall bladder—Yang

The Six Meridians Located in the Arms

Li	Large intestine—Yang
Si	Small intestine—Yang
Ht	Heart—Yin
Pc	Pericardium—protects the heart—Yin
TW	Triple Warmer—abdominal—Yang
Lu	Lung—Yin

Notice that the Yin (female) meridians primarily relate to the life support of the person and the Yang (male) meridians primarily relate to the digestive system.

Chi and Meridians

The only two meridians (vessels) that do not have pairs are the Governing Vessel and the Conception Vessel.

GV Governing Vessel   (Yang) from the tail-bone up the back and over the head, to the center of the upper lip.

CV Conception Vessel   (Yin) from the perineum up the center of the abdomen and chest, and up to the center of the lower lip.

Each meridian serves a specific part of the body. The pressure points on a specific meridian will relate to its function. They are identified by a letter or letters, indicating the meridian; and a number, indicating the location on that meridian.

For example, Kd6 is pressure point number 6 on the Kidney meridian. Located near the ankle, this pressure point is named Shining Sea. Pressing this point sends Yin energy up the Kidney meridian to the throat, providing moisture and coolness to a sore throat.

Although the Governing Vessel runs upward from the tailbone, over the head and down to the upper lip, it is still a Yang meridian. The Conception Vessel runs from the perineum up the abdomen, across the center of the chest to the lower lip.

Chi and Meridians

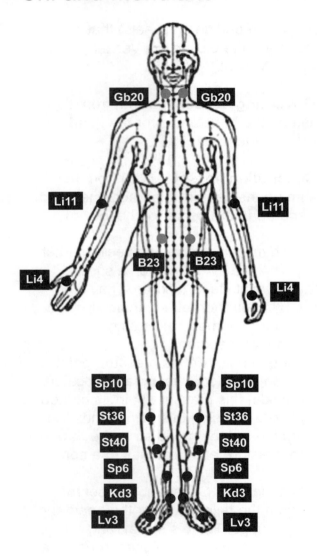

Chi and Meridians

The picture on the preceding page can be intimidating, so let's examine it in small increments. Each of the arms and legs has six meridians. However, for simplicity, we only illustrate the ten primary pressure points. As we learned earlier, every meridian has a mirror meridian on the opposite side of the body. The two exceptions are the Governing Vessel, Yang (male) and the Conception Vessel, Yin (female) which are located on the midline of the body. The ten primary points are pictured in pairs.

As you will learn, some pressure points are used more frequently than other points; they have more healing power than other minor points. The direction of the meridian numbers will indicate the gender of the meridian, Yin (female) or Yang (male). With arms raised over the head, the meridian numbers decrease or increase from top downward. When the numbers decrease, this is a Yin meridian, and when the numbers increase this is a Yang meridian. This is apparent for the leg meridians, but may be confusing for the arm meridians.

The anatomical position for the human body in Eastern cultures is arms raised over the head. If we raise our arms over our head, all the numbers are in the correct direction.

Chi and Meridians

The Governing and the Conception Vessels are located on the midline of the body. The Governing Vessel (male) runs up the back, over the head, and down to the upper lip. The Conception Vessel (female) runs from the perineum, over the abdomen, and up to the lower lip. The Yang meridians refer to functions of nutrition and digestion, and the Yin meridians refer to reproductive and sexual functions and to life support.

With arms over the head, the Eastern anatomical position, the meridian numbers increasing up the arms are the Yin (female) meridians, and the numbers increasing down the arms belong to Yang (male) meridians.

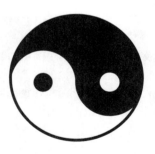

Acupressure

Acupressure is about two thousand years older than acupuncture. This practice of using fingers and thumbs to activate pressure points is estimated to be about five thousand years old. Acupressure is the practice of locating and releasing blocked or congested energy centers in the body. It is relatively easy to learn and practice. Unlike acupuncture, where a practitioner inserts a needle, you simply apply pressure usually with your thumb to the relevant acupressure point. The same pressure points are used with both acupressure and acupuncture.

Acupressure is believed to originate in China, but two major cultures, Chinese and Japanese, have refined this practice. The Chinese discovered the healing properties of pressure points, and the Japanese identified specific pathways of these pressure points. These pathways were described as "meridians" that indicated specific directions and flow of the energy Chi. The Japanese identified these meridians about three thousand years ago. Recent electronic imaging has identified the pathways of the human neurology. The result was that these pathways and the ancient meridians are almost identical. It is an amazing to realize that the Japanese were so accurate in identifying these pathways so long ago.

Acupressure

A meridian has a beginning, an end, and various points along the way where problems can develop. Along the meridians these points are specific locations allowing energy to flow before moving to the next point on the meridian. If a point becomes constricted, energy cannot flow in a normal pattern. The purpose of acupressure is to normalize the energy flow and return the body to a healthy state.

Acupressure can successfully treat common conditions, such as anxiety, stress, insomnia, indigestion, aches and pains, headaches and migraine, fatigue and many more. Because the benefits are fast and the side effects are virtually nonexistent, this natural practice continues to be one of the most popular in the world.

The best way to learn acupressure is to practice. Practicing on yourself can give you a good sense of how these points can relate to different symptoms.

How to Find
a Pressure Point.

Although there are over 350 pressure points in the human body, only a few are primary points. Most are referred to as "helper points." We will focus on the primary points for the fastest relief.

Let's locate a primary pressure point that is easy to find. Tilt your head forward and place the middle fingers of both your hands on the back of your neck. Find the base of your skull and feel the small depression in the center or the midline of the base. Move your fingers away from the center along the base about one inch to either side. You have located the Gb20 pressure points also known as Wind Pool. These two points are on the Gallbladder (Gb) meridian; they are pressure points number 20. Massaging these pressure points for up to one minute with mild to moderate pressure will reduce stress, neck stiffness, headache pain, and cold symptoms.

You will read the terms "mild" or "moderate" when applying pressure. This is where the amount of pressure becomes personalized. Pressure needs to be exerted in order to activate the pressure point. Properly applying pressure is important for maximum effect of acupressure.

How to Find
a Pressure Point.

To find a pressure point, you will have to press with enough firmness to feel the sensitivity or tingling from that point. Once you have found the point, increase the pressure ever so slightly. If you can feel a gentle warmth radiating from the point, you are doing it correctly. If you feel pain radiating, you are pressing too heavily. If you feel little or no sensation, you will need to press a little firmer. Remember that some of these pressure points are more sensitive than others, so quality of pressure will be important to adjust from point to point. Some pressure points require pressure without massage and are indicated with a notation of PRESS ONLY.

      The key to pressure is effectiveness. Do not press too hard to experience pain. However, you do want to press and massage each point with enough pressure to activate the point for healing benefits. Remember that pressing a point is not only stimulating circulation, it is stimulates the nervous system at the same time.

IMPORTANT! Remember to press right and left pressure points at the same time. Pressure points are illustrated from head to toe for reference only and not a sequence for treatment. Each person should discover the most effective pressure points for treatments.

Hand
Positions

There are four hand positions commonly used in acupressure. It is important to use the hand positions that do not cause excessive joint stress or pressure.

1. Pad of the Thumb. This hand position is by far the most common technique. Using this technique may feel unusual and require some practice.

2. Pad of the Index Finger. This hand position is used for direct pressure on small areas. Pressure can be increased by overlapping the middle finger over the nail of the index finger.

3. Tips of the Index, Middle, and Ring Fingers. This hand position is commonly used for larger pressure areas when additional pressure is indicated.

4. MCP Joint (the large knuckle of middle finger). This hand position is used for large muscle discomfort, such as in the lower back.

Remember to protect your hands and joints from excessive stress and pressure. Acupressure therapists have traditionally used the thumbs when applying pressure, but years of practice have resulted in variations. They also use elbows, forearms, even feet to activate pressure points.

Hand
Positions

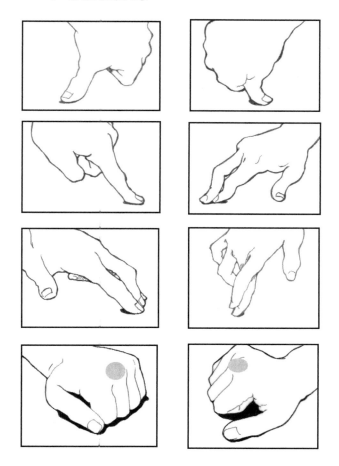

Rules for Using Acupressure

Breathe from your diaphragm. Inhale through your nose, exhale from your mouth.

Do not perform acupressure if you have taken pain medication.

Do not drink alcoholic beverages before self-treatment.

Stop self-treatment if you experience pain.

Do not treat areas that are injured or have open cuts, sunburn, infections, or skin disorders.

For acute symptoms, you can apply pressure point treatment for up to three times daily.

Apply pressure to an acupressure point for up to one minute using a massaging motion.

The location of pressure points may slightly vary in each person. Locate each of the points and practice until you can find them without looking.

Do not let acupressure replace other treatment that your physician or healthcare professional feels is necessary.

Aromatherapy -

The Egyptians practiced a process called "infusion," the process of making essences and oils from plants. This practice is common today in preparing teas which, once ingested, are quickly absorbed into the system. Because they are liquids, benefits from these teas can be felt almost immediately. Note that not all essences and oils can be taken internally, so seek the advice of an herbologist and follow the instructions given by the manufacturer.

The first use of infusions was for aromatic purposes. The Egyptians burned common essences of Myrrh and Frankincense burned as incense for celebrating and honoring their gods. In the ritual of embalming, oils were used for preserving and mummifying the bodies of the dead. In addition, Egyptians and Greeks used oils for massage and for their healing properties. The Greeks actually documented the use and purpose of using oils as a curative practice. Their records became the standard for practice by Western cultures for over one thousand years. Some historians believe the Chinese were using essences and oils about the same time as the Egyptians. Aromatherapy has become popular in Western cultures in the recent years,

Aromatherapy

and the practice is receiving attention as an important part of alternative medicine.

Aromatherapy has gained importance due to its effect on the limbic system. The limbic system directly connects to the areas of the brain that affect heart rate, respiration, memory, stress level, and hormone balance. More specifically, the olfactory nerve, when stimulated by aromatherapy, influences the limbic system in a positive way. When the limbic system calms and relaxes the mind and body, this lowers stress, anxiety, nervousness, muscle tension, and fatigue. The body is then in a relaxed state, and therapies, such as acupressure and herbal therapy, can have a more positive effect on health and wellness.

As a general rule in this book, all essences are classified into two areas. For aromatherapy, they can either be inhaled or applied directly to the skin. Nearly all of these essences oils can be purchased and kept in small bottles. Follow the directions on the packages or seek information from a qualified practitioner or professional. For professional assistance, purchase essences and oils from a seller who knows the products and contents. Health food stores are an excellent resource for quality aromatherapy products and professional support. The staff are knowledgeable and helpful in recommending

Aromatherapy

products and proper usage for the most effective results.

Many of these essences and oils can be purchased at health food stores, such as Whole Foods Markets. Essences and oils usually are sold in concentrated form and should be diluted. Essences and oils applied full strength to the skin, such as clove, can cause an irritation or rash.

HELPFUL HINTS
Studies have shown that Ginger can be up to three times more effective preventing motion sickness and nausea than over-the-counter medications.

The word tincture refers to alcohol. If you have adverse reactions to alcohol, make sure the oils do not contain it.

For a complete list of aromas positively affecting conditions and ailments, refer to *Appendix A* at the back of this book.

Herbology.

Four separate and distinct geographic areas understood and practiced herbology. Each culture was separated by thousands of miles, and some by oceans, yet each developed a sophisticated practice of herbology with strong similarities to each other: the Middle East, India, China/Japan, and Greece/Italy.

Middle East herbal practice dates back to the Mesopotamian and Egyptian civilizations 1,500 to 2,000 B.C. Greek and Roman herbal practices, from written work, date back to the first century A.D. Indian culture developed Ayurvedic medicine which emerged during the development of the Upanishads, Buddhism, and other schools of thought in India. Herbs have played an important role in Ayurvedic medicine for some 2,000 years. The earliest written evidence of the medicinal use of herbs in China consists of a corpus of 11 medical works recovered from a burial site in Hunan province. The estimated date of earliest Chinese practice is about 300 B.C. Traditional Chinese medicine was brought to Japan via Korea, and Chinese-influenced Korean medicine was adapted by the Japanese during the reign of Emperor Ingyo 411-453 A.D. These cultures influenced the growth and expansion of herbal medicine.

Herbology

Today The World Health Organization (WHO) estimates that 5 billion people, 80 percent of the world population, use herbal medicine for some aspect of primary health care. Nearly every country in the world uses some form of herbal medicine for ailments and medical conditions. Because of the popularity of herbal medicine, new and effective herbal treatments are being offered to those seeking alternative approaches for natural health.

In the United States, the American Botanical Council is an excellent resource for current information on research and information about herbal medicine. This includes current news, trends, and studies on herbal medicine.

Herbs in the home are very common. Nearly everyone has several around the kitchen, such as cinnamon, garlic, pepper, and ginger. All four of these have specific properties for health and wellness.

Before starting an herbal therapy program, consult with a certified herbologist. If you are taking prescription medications, inform your physician that you are considering herbal therapy. If you need assistance with herbs, I again recommend Whole Foods Markets. The staff is very knowledgeable and can assist with developing a customized herbal program.

Twelve Common Herbs

This section is a brief introduction to the properties of some common herbs. If you decide to try herbal medicine, it is very important to read, study, and seek professional information and advice before starting herbal therapy. Many common herbs that are safe for animals are toxic, even fatal, to humans.

How do herbs work? Traditional medicines direct a medication's properties to a specific site or problem in the body. Herbs, in contrast, work to help strengthen the body by effectively buffering and supporting the immune system and the healing process. Peppermint, for example, aids digestion, cleanses bad breath, reduces upset stomach, and is a mild decongestant.

The medicinal part of an herb may be the leaf, flower, fruit, stem, bark, or root. Herbs may be used in a variety of ways, such as whole form, capsules, tablets, teas, syrups, ointments, oils, and compresses. One of the most common ways to take herbs is by *infusion,* or brewed as a tea. Tea is a very pleasant way to ingest the herb, and, since it has a water-soluble base, tea is quickly absorbed into the body.

Organically grown herbs have greater purity than those grown non-organically.

Twelve Common Herbs

Fresh herbs have a more positive effect on the body. Although some herbs require preparation, such as drying, most fresh, organic herbs have a higher potency and purity than commercially prepared herbs.

Herbal mixtures and elixers contain more than one kind of herb and different amounts of herbs. Sometimes the name on the bottle or container does not describe its content, so seeking the advice of a qualified professional is important to assure that the herbal mixture or elixer is beneficial for you. Unless you grow and process your own herbs, professional guidance is essential for maximum safety and benefits. Read and follow all instructions and precautions included with any commercially prepared products.

IMPORTANT!
Some of the herbs that may cause adverse effects are the following:
angelica, bayberry, black cohosh, ephedra, fenugreek, shepherd's purse, tea tree, and vervain.

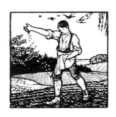

1. Cat's claw

This plant, also called Una de Gato, is a tropical vine that comes from the Peruvian Amazon. It is a relative to the coffee plant. The plant's bark is used in herbal therapy.

WHAT IT DOES
The bark is rich in sterols, a chemical compound resembling steroids, is an anti-inflammatory, aids the immune system.

FOR THESE CONDITIONS
Arthritis, bowel disorders, peptic ulcers, gastritis, colds, Lyme disease.

PRECAUTIONS
People who are insulin dependent, pregnant women, and nursing mothers.

METHOD AND DOSAGE
Cat's claw can be taken by capsule or in *tincture* form. Remember *tincture* means alcohol. Cat's claw should be taken with an 8 oz. glass of water and adding a teaspoon of lemon juice or vinegar.

2. Chamomile

This herb has the appearance of a small daisy with feathery leaves and a distinctive smell. The two most common types are German chamomile and garden chamomile.

WHAT IT DOES
The herb is an anti-inflammatory, antioxidant, and an antiseptic. Chamomile inhibits the growth of underarm bacteria.

FOR THESE CONDITIONS
Allergies, asthma, anxiety, cuts, scrapes, abrasions, peptic ulcers, and premenstrual symptoms.

PRECAUTIONS
None.

METHOD AND DOSAGE
Chamomile comes in forms of teas and tinctures for internal use and creams for external use. This herb has an accumulative effect, so results may not be noticed for several weeks.

3. Cinnamon

Although we think of cinnamon as a spice, it is an herb with medicinal properties. This herb is the bark or twigs of a tree that is commonly grown in India, Sri Lanka, and the West Indies.

WHAT IT DOES
Aids digestion, is an antiseptic,
an antispasmodic, and is a gentle stimulant.

FOR THESE CONDITIONS
Colds, fever, indigestion, peptic ulcer,
menstrual problems, and yeast infections.

PRECAUTIONS
None.

METHOD AND DOSAGE
Cinnamon can be purchased as an oil,
sticks called *quills,* or as a ground powder.
Place one inch of the quill or full pinch in
8 oz. of hot water. It makes this a tasty tea
for colds and fever. Adding about ten drops of
the oil to eight oz. of warm water will aid
digestion and calm nervous stomachs.

4. Comfrey

Comfrey is a large-leaf plant that grows well in temperate climates. The flowers can be white, pink, or purple in color, and the flowers, leaves, and stems are used in herbal therapy. The roots are toxic.

WHAT IT DOES
Relieves pain and inflammation due to injury and muscular degeneration.

FOR THESE CONDITIONS
Wounds, cuts, sprains, and arthritis. Internally, stomach ulcers, indigestion, and coughs.

PRECAUTIONS
Pregnant women and nursing mothers.

METHOD AND DOSAGE
Externally as a cream or salve, or as a compress applied to the skin. Internally as a tea for stomach ulcers and indigestion and as a syrup for dry coughs.

5. Ginger

Ginger is probably the most widely used herb in the world. The plant grows about two feet high with sharp pointed leaves and white or yellow flowers. The medicinal part of this tropical plant is the root, also referred to as the *tuber*. It is also used as a common kitchen spice.

WHAT IT DOES
Promotes cleansing of the body, reduce pain and inflammation, and is an antispasmodic.

FOR THESE CONDITIONS
Nausea, travel sickness, upset stomach, nausea from pregnancy, poor appetite, menstrual pains, chills, and hiccups.

PRECAUTIONS
None.

METHOD AND DOSAGE
Ten to fifteen drops of tincture in tea or mixed in a teaspoon of honey. Use grated root made into a tea for chills and nausea. Also candied and in capsules for upset stomach and nausea.

6. Hawthorn

The Hawthorn tree is a member of the rose family and commonly seen in parks and gardens. Spring's white flowers turn to berries in the summer. Both are used in herbal therapy.

WHAT IT DOES
Heart and circulatory restorative, lowers blood pressure, recovery from heart attack.

FOR THESE CONDITIONS
Strengthens heart muscle and circulation, treatment for Alzheimer's disease and memory loss, high blood pressure, angina, arrhythmia, atherosclerosis, arthritis, and ADD.

PRECAUTIONS
Heart disease should be treated by a professional.

METHOD AND DOSAGE
Three to four teaspoons of tincture daily for six months. Take capsules and tablets as directed.

7. Kava

Kava is an evergreen shrub that is native to the South Pacific islands and can grow up to ten feet in height. It has a soft stem and heart-shaped leaves. The dried root is used in herbal therapy.

WHAT IT DOES
Kava is a sedative, analgesic, antiseptic, and mild euphoriant. The sedative property has a calming effect without impairing mental clarity.

FOR THESE CONDITIONS
Mild anxiety and depression, insomnia, and toothache. The analgesic properties are also used for kidney and urinary track discomfort.

PRECAUTIONS
Not to be taken with prescription medications for depression or anxiety or by pregnant women and people on psychotropic medications.

METHOD AND DOSAGE
Kava is taken as directed in tablet form, and tablets should contain 70% kavalactones.

8. Lavender

Lavender is a low-growing shrub that is native to Mediterranean countries, but has been a favorite in English gardens. Today it is commonly grown in North America. The shrub has multiple stems with spikes of purple flowers. The flowers are used in herbal therapy.

WHAT IT DOES
Lavender has been used as a sedative, diuretic, antispasmodic, and digestive aid.

FOR THESE CONDITIONS
Common remedy for ailments of headache, insomnia, nausea, nervousness, fatigue, and skin conditions of acne, psoriasis, and fungal conditions.

PRECAUTIONS
Do not take lavender oil internally.

METHOD AND DOSAGE
Lavender oil may be used in compresses, baths, and products, such as soaps and lotions, or applied directly to the skin. Lavender is also a very popular and soothing oil in aromatherapy.

9. Lemon balm

Lemon balm is commonly grown in many Mediterranean countries. A member of the mint family, it has leaves in pairs with white flowers. The flowers are primarily used in herbal therapy, but today the leaves and stems are also used for their medicinal properties.

WHAT IT DOES
The herb is a mild sedative, a mild antibacterial and antiviral, and antidepressant.

FOR THESE CONDITIONS
Indigestion, depression, nervousness, insomnia, stress, irritable bowel syndrome, and Herpes infection.

PRECAUTIONS
Pregnant or lactating women should not use this herb.

METHOD AND DOSAGE
Lemon balm is available in creams for topical treatment of skin disorders, or tablets, oils, and teas for internal use. This herb is mild enough for infants and children.

10. Saw palmetto

Saw Palmetto is a small, palm-like plant native to North America. Native Americans and early American settlers used the berries to treat problems associated with the genitals, urinary tract and reproductive system. Saw Palmetto is now used in the U.S. for nutritionally benefiting the prostate and urinary tract. It has been marketed as an aphrodisiac for both men and women.

WHAT IT DOES
Saw palmetto inhibits androgen and estrogen receptor activity and may be beneficial for both sexes in balancing hormones.

FOR THESE CONDITIONS
For men, it treats an enlarged and weakened prostate gland. Women have used the herb to stimulate breast enlargement and lactation as well as treating ovarian and uterine irritability.

PRECAUTIONS
Pregnant women should not use this herb.

METHOD AND DOSAGE
Fresh berries and dried berries as capsules or in preparation as a tincture.

11. St. John's wort

St. John's wort is native to Great Britain, particularly Wales. *Wort* refers to any plant that is used for medicinal purposes. This small tree grows up to three feet with clusters of yellow flowers that bloom around St. John's Day. The entire tree is used for herbal therapy.

WHAT IT DOES
Antibacterial, antidepressant, antiviral, pain reliever.

FOR THESE CONDITIONS
In addition to fighting depression, the herb is also used for treating fatigue, Lyme disease, relieving throat pain, and headaches, nasal congestion, cuts and scrapes.

PRECAUTIONS
Avoid excessive direct sunlight exposure.

METHOD AND DOSAGE
This herb may be taken as a tea, one to two 8 oz. cups daily or tincture, three to four teaspoons daily, and tablets and capsules as directed.

12. Yarrow

Yarrow is a weed-like plant with feathery leaves and white or pink flowers. This plant grows up to three feet high, and the flowers, leaves, and stems are used in herbal treatment. Greek legend says that Achilles used yarrow to stop the bleeding of his soldiers.

WHAT IT DOES
Anti-inflammatory, diaphoretic, antispasmodic, strengthens peripheral circulation.

FOR THESE CONDITIONS
Healing of cuts and bruises, relieves cramps and other menstrual pain, reduces insomnia, reduces fever, diarrhea, and stomach cramps.

PRECAUTIONS
Avoid large doses during pregnancy, clean cuts and bruises thoroughly before applying to the skin. Topical treatment may cause skin irritation. Avoid if experiencing gallstones.

METHOD AND DOSAGE
As a tea, three 8 oz.cups a day to strengthen circulation; as a topical treatment.

Ten Primary Pressure Points

In this section we will describe and locate and apply pressure to ten of the primary pressure points of the body. This is an exercise to practice locating and activating pressure points. Once you can effectively use these ten points, you can easily continue to the most important section of this book: self-treating ailments and conditions. Most of these points influence the flow and intensity of the energy, or Chi, within us. Opening or releasing the blocks in these points will increase our well-being and general health. They can also be used to relieve particular symptoms.

You will notice throughout this book that many of the primary pressure points are used to help more than one condition. Because of their healing power they can, along with other helping pressure points, contribute to the effectiveness of your treatment. Most pressure points are associated with specific conditions, but these primary points can also contribute to general good health.

IMPORTANT!
Please note any precautions. Several pressure points have serious cautions for people with certain conditions.

Ten Primary Pressure Points

Of more than 350 pressure points in the body, ten are considered the most influential and powerful. By far referred to as the Ten Primary Pressure Points because of their significance, they will be the best first-aid kit you will ever have!

Gb20 Wind Pool (base of the skull).
Li11 Pool at the Crook (bend of the elbow).
Li4 Adjoining Valley (web of the hand).
B23 Associated Point of Kidney (lower back).
Sp10 Sea of Blood (three inches above the knee).
St36 Three Mile Foot (three inches below knee).
St40 Abundant Splendor (beside shin bone).
Sp6 Three Yin Meeting (above ankle bone).
Kd3 Supreme Stream (behind ankle bone).
Lv3 Bigger Rushing (top of foot).

If you remember the Meridians, these initials will be familiar. What colorful names the Chinese gave to such powerful pressure points! Ancient practitioners understood the importance of their healing power.

Gb20
Wind Pool

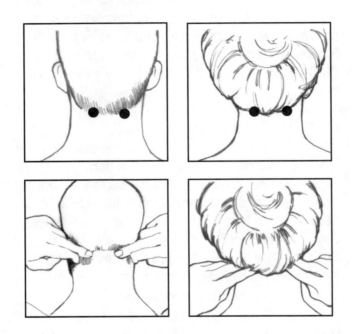

Gb20
Wind Pool

Treatment

Headaches.

Colds.

Stiffness.

Place the fingers of both hands just at the base of the skull. Feel the depression at the base. Move the fingers along the base and away from the spine about one inch on either side. With your thumbs or fingers massage these points with moderate pressure for up to one minute.

Though not one of the primary pressure points, GV16 called Naohu, Doorway to the Brain, is located at the center of the base of the skull. Feel for the depression and massage this area with your thumb or middle and ring fingers. This pressure point stimulates oxygen to the brain and increases attention and concentration.

Li11
Pool at the Crook

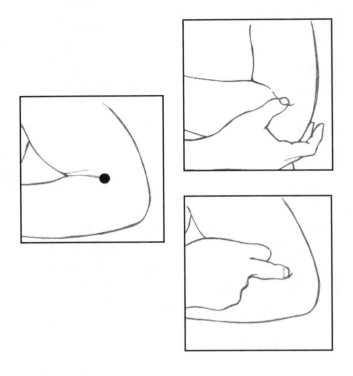

Li11
Pool at the Crook

Treatment
Relieves pain in the arm.
Regulates intestinal anxiety.
Helps to eliminate excess heat and moisture from the body (fever).

To find this pressure point, hold your hand over your heart. Notice the crease at your elbow. At the outside of the crease is the Pool at the Crook. Use your thumb or finger to apply a massaging pressure for up to one minute. Apply pressure for the same amount of time to the other arm. This pressure point may take a little practice to locate, but is well worth the benefits.

When applying pressure to any of the meridian pressure points, be sure to apply equal pressure to the same pressure point on the opposite side. This is important to keep the balance of energy within the body.

Li4
Adjoining Valley

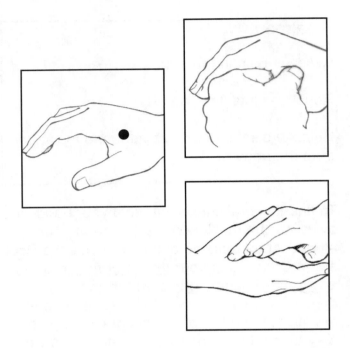

Li4
Adjoining Valley

Treatment
Headaches.
Pain.
Muscular tension.
Clears excess heat from the body (fever).

This pressure point is located near the web of the hand between the index finger and the thumb. Locate the large muscle in the web area and press to locate this point. The best technique is to use the index finger and the thumb. Hold this point for up to one minute and repeat on the other hand.

CAUTION! Women who are pregnant should not use this pressure point. Activating this pressure point can cause contractions of the uterus.

B23
Associated Point of Kidney

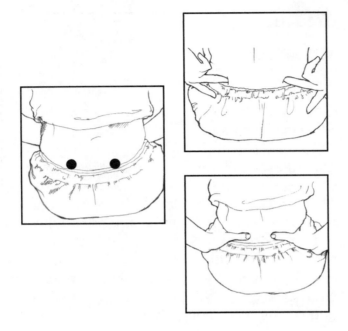

B23
Associated Point of Kidney

Treatment
Stress.
Aids in the flow of Chi in the body.
Low back pain.

This pressure point is located about two inches on either side of the spine. Trace a path from the navel around to the back. This pressure point is located just below that path. To apply pressure to these points, use your thumbs or middle fingers. This is also a good time to use the large knuckle of the middle finger with the hand in a fist position. Another suggestion is to tie two tennis balls in a sock and place the sock against the back of your chair or against a wall. Apply pressure to these points for up to one minute.

Sp10
Sea of Blood

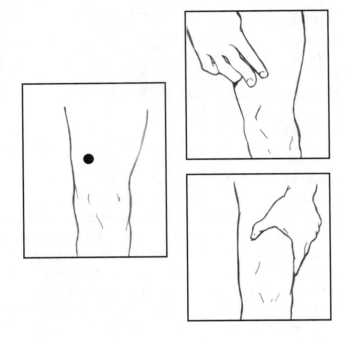

Sp10
Sea of Blood

Treatment

Stagnation of fluids in the abdominal area.

Aids in healing and nourishing of the skin.

Locate this pressure point about three inches above the knee and about one inch to the inside. This point is located on the large teardrop shaped muscle of the upper leg. Use either thumb pressure or pressure from the knuckle of the middle finger. Apply pressure for up to one minute. Apply pressure to both legs or one at a time.

When locating and treating pressure points over muscular areas of the body, you will need to apply more pressure. Areas that are more superficial, such as the face, ankles, and feet, require less pressure. Adjust the intensity of pressure, but keep the one minute time for each point.

St36
Three Mile Foot

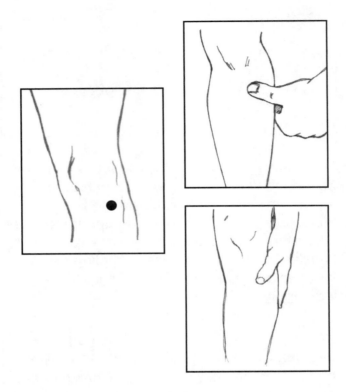

St36
Three Mile Foot

Treatment

Revitalizes Chi and fluids of the entire body.

Increases energy and stamina.

This point is located about three inches below the knee cap and in the depression just to the outside of the shin bone. Use your index or middle finger to apply massaging pressure to this point for up to one minute. This pressure point is most effective when pressure is applied to both legs at the same time. Apply light to medium pressure with a massaging motion.

A "shin splint" is a soft tissue tear that runners often experience in the front of the leg. These shin splints often occur around the location of the Three Mile Foot. Soft tissue injuries can often take longer to heal than a bone fracture.

St40
Abundant Splendor

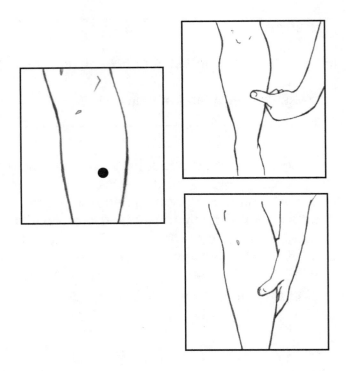

St40
Abundant Splendor

Treatment
Eliminates congestion.
Reduces mucus.
Increases respiration.

Location of this pressure point is half-way between the knee and the ankle about one and one-half inches to the outside of the shin bone. This pressure point can be started with light pressure and increased to moderate since it is located within a large muscle. The most effective pressure is with the index or middle finger for up to one minute on each point. Congestion can refer to symptoms from colds, allergies, and flu.

Sp6
Three Yin Meeting

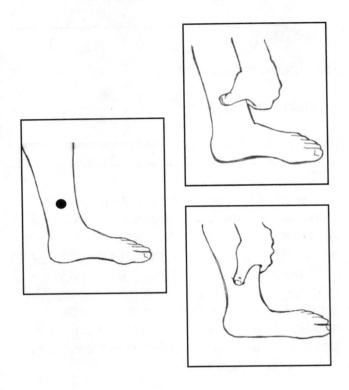

Sp6
Three Yin Meeting

Treatment
Menstrual cramps.
Menopause.
Enhances the flow of Chi throughout the body.

This is one of the most important pressure points of the body, because it is the meeting of three female meridians: Kidney, Liver, and Spleen. Locate this point on the inside of the lower leg about three inches above the ankle bone and one-half inch toward the back of the leg. <u>Use your index finger or thumb to apply pressure for up to one minute to each point.</u>

CAUTION! Women who are pregnant should not use this pressure point. Activating this pressure point can cause contractions of the uterus.

Kd3
Supreme Stream

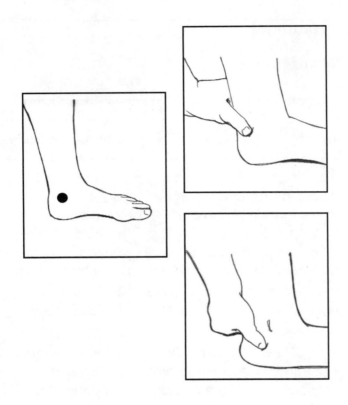

Kd3
Supreme Stream

> **Treatment**
>
> Energizes and detoxifies the body.
>
> Impotence.
>
> Kidney function.

This pressure point can be easily located. It lies between the inside ankle bone and the Achilles tendon or heel cord. With your thumb, feel for the depression between the ankle bone and heel cord and begin with mild pressure in a massaging motion with your thumb for up to one minute. Unless you are very limber, you may need to massage one ankle at a time.

> Chinese medicine considers this pressure point one of the most important points of the body. It stimulates the Kidney Chi, which has the most powerful effect on Yin and Yang.

Lv3
Bigger Rushing

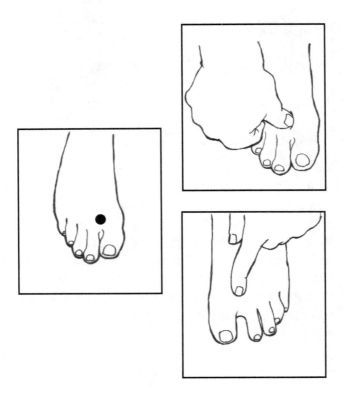

Lv3
Bigger Rushing

Treatment

Excellent reliever of stress.

Aids the circulation of Chi.

Menstrual difficulties.

This point is located on top of the foot between the tendons of the great and second toes. To locate this point, place your finger in the web between the toes and draw the finger toward the ankle about one-half to one inch. This will be the location of the pressure point. Press and massage gently up to one minute, because this point is close to the surface and may be sensitive.

This point is most effective when pressing both feet with the index fingers or thumbs simultaneously. If you have difficulty reaching your feet, take off your shoes and use your heel to massage the Bigger Rushing on the other foot. Notice the two different pressure techniques.

Common Conditions
and Treatments

The ten primary points gave you a frame of reference for locating and using pressure points. Finding the correct amount of pressure is a developed skill that takes a little practice, but is well worth the time. The results will be excellent.

This section of the book covers ailments or conditions that you might experience on the job, in a classroom, at home, or when traveling. There are over one hundred conditions that acupressure, herbal remedies, and aromatherapy may help alleviate. Here we will cover the most common conditions. As many as twenty pressure points can help a particular condition. However, only the key points will be listed here. That will make it easier for you to remember them.

Pressure points from different meridians or vessels are often used when treating the same condition. This illustrates the healing power of points from other meridians for treating a condition or ailment.

You will also notice that some of the primary pressure points may appear frequently here for different conditions. Look for the * symbol next to these pressure points. This is a reminder of their importance and enormous healing power.

Common Conditions
and Treatments

The following section also contains
suggestions for using aromatherapy and
herbal therapy when treating the conditions.
Helpful herbs are listed in alphabetical order
for reference only, but herbs in **bold print** are
described in the section titled <u>Twelve Common
Herbs</u>.

IMPORTANT!
Any herbal therapy should be under the
advice of a qualified professional. A
credentialed herbologist can provide important
information. If you are taking prescribed
medications, consult your physician before
taking herbs.

When conducting acupressure treatments,
press right and left side pressure points at the
same time.

Allergies, Congestion

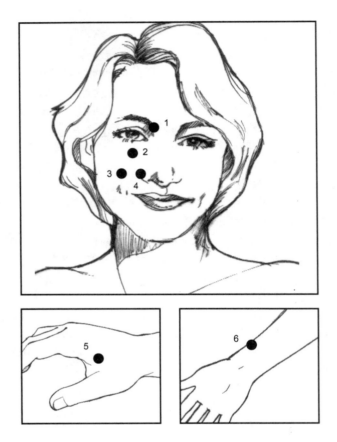

Allergies encompass a wide range of symptoms. The severity of allergic reactions can depend on the allergen type, the level of exposure and the individual's response. Common symptoms are watery, itchy eyes, sneezing, scratchy throat, headache, hives, tiredness, and sinusitis.

Allergies, Congestion

PRESSURE POINTS
1. B2 On the inside corner of the eyebrow.
PRESS ONLY

2. St1 Below the center of the eye.

3. Si18 Below the cheekbone.

4. Li20 Beside the corner of the nose.
PRESS ONLY

5. Li4* Web of the hand.

6. Lu7 Two inches above the wrist
on the thumb side.

AROMATHERAPY
Chamomile

HELPFUL HERBS
Chamomile, **Ginger**, Peppermint.

CAUTION! Women who are pregnant should
not use pressure point Li4.

*Allergies to peanut and tree nuts, such as
pecans, walnuts, almonds, can be a serious
condition. These affect approximately three
million Americans. Peanuts are the leading
cause of severe food allergic reactions,
followed by shellfish, fish, tree nuts and eggs.*

Angina

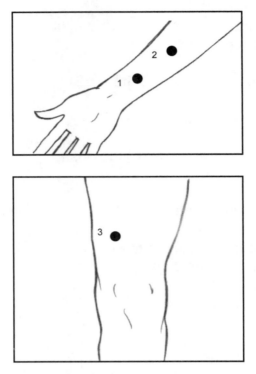

Angina, a condition of coronary artery disease, is chest pain or discomfort that occurs when your heart muscle does not get enough blood. Symptoms may include pressure or a squeezing pain in the chest. The pain may also occur in the arms, neck, jaw, shoulders, or back. It may also feel like indigestion. This is a condition that requires immediate medical attention.

Angina

PRESSURE POINTS
1. **Pc6** About two inches above the wrist in the center of the palm side forearm.

2. **Pc4** Located half way between the wrist and elbow.

3. **Sp10*** Sea of Blood, three inches above the knee.

AROMATHERAPY
Ginger.

HELPFUL HERBS
Astragalus, **hawthorn.**

CAUTION! This is not a condition to be taken lightly. Medical attention should be sought immediately.

To have your "heart in your mouth" means that you are frightened or anxious about something. The ancient Greek poet Homer used the phrase thousands of years ago when he wrote the famous poem "The Iliad," and people have been using it ever since. When your heart starts pounding so much that you can feel a thumping in your throat, it may feel like you "have your heart in your mouth."

Anxiety, Nervousness

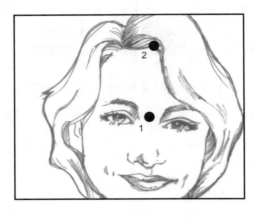

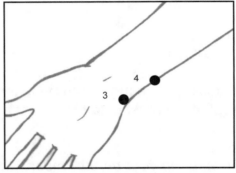

People of all ages are affected by general anxiety disorder. Anxiety is twice as likely to appear in women as in men. Symptoms can appear in childhood and adolescence. Research suggests that environmental and genetic factors, such as family history of anxiety, may predispose a person to develop the disorder.

Anxiety, Nervousness

PRESSURE POINTS
1. **Yin Tang** On the bridge of the nose between the eyebrows. PRESS ONLY

2. **GV24** Just at the hairline in the center of the head. PRESS ONLY

3. **Ht7** Located on the side of your wrist in the indentation on the little finger side.

4. **Ht5** About two inches above the crease of the wrist.

AROMATHERAPY
Lavender, orange blossom, tangerine.

HELPFUL HERBS
Chamomile, **ginger**, ginseng, **kava**, passionflower, **St. John's wort**, valerian.

"Butterflies in the stomach" is a way of describing nervous, fluttery feelings you might have before a major event. An imaginative writer created the phrase to describe the feeling, and people have been using it ever since. Some people believe having a few butterflies might even help you perform better by keeping you alert and on your toes.

Arthritis

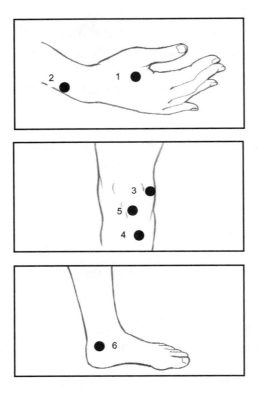

Osteoarthritis usually occurs in the large joints, such as shoulders and hips, and spine of the body causing bony parts to rub together because of cartilage deterioration. Rheumatoid arthritis is most common in the wrists, ankles, hands, and feet causing joint deterioration and deformity. Osteoarthritis usually occurs in later years; RA can occur in early childhood.

Arthritis

PRESSURE POINTS
1. **Li4*** Web of the hand.
   (Point for Rheumatoid Arthritis)

2. **TW5** Two inches above the wrist on the back of the arm.

3. **St35** On the outside of the knee joint.

4. **St36*** Three inches below the knee beside the shin bone.

5. **Gb41** Lower border of the knee cap.

6. **Kd3*** Inside of the foot between the ankle and Achilles tendon.

AROMATHERAPY
Eucalyptus, juniper.

HELPFUL HERBS
OSTEOARTHRITIS:
Cat's claw, cayenne, **comfrey**, **ginger**, **hawthorn**, willow bark.
RHEUMATOID ARTHRITIS:
Cat's claw, **comfrey**, **hawthorn**.

People suffering with arthritis may prefer a cold wrap instead of a warm wrap applied to an arthritic joint for pain relief.

Asthma

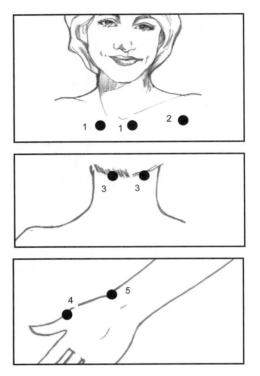

Asthma is very common among children, teens and adults. It is a disease that causes the airways of the lungs to tighten. An asthma attack occurs when the lungs are not getting enough air to breathe. Symptoms of an asthma attack may be trouble breathing, wheezing. coughing, chest pain, and chest tightness. Asthma can be triggered by mold, dust mites, secondhand smoke, cats and dogs.

Asthma

PRESSURE POINTS
1. **Kd27** Two inches either side of the
   sternum under the collar bone.

2. **Lu1** In the shoulder depression about two
   inches below the collar bone.

3. **B13** Tilt your head forward and feel the
   bump about four inches below the
   center of the skull base. This point is
   about two inches down and one inch
   either side of the spine.

4. **Lu10** In the center of the thumb between
   the first and second joints.

5. **Lv9** In the fold of the wrist below the
   thumb.

AROMATHERAPY
Coffee, eucalyptus.

HELPFUL HERBS
Chamomile, elderberry, **ginger**, green tea,
licorice,

*Sipping hot coffee seems to bring fast relief
from an asthmatic attack. The heat and coffee
aromatic properties appear to relax bronchial
spasms.*

Back Pain

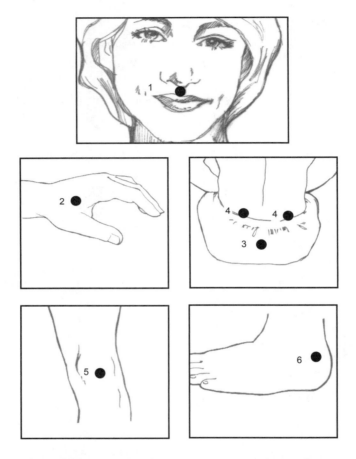

Back pain is a term that covers a variety of upper, middle, and lower back discomforts. The causes of back pain can be related to muscular, skeletal, or neurological problems. These pressure points are commonly used in treatments by healthcare professionals.

Back Pain

PRESSURE POINTS
1. GV25 Between the upper lip and nose.
 PRESS ONLY

2. Li4* Web of the hand.

3. GV2 At the fold of the buttocks between
 the sacrum and coccyx.

4. B23* About two inches either side of the
 spine. For best effect, massage these
 two points at the same time.

5. B40 Back of the knee in the crease
 between the two large tendons.

6. B60 Between the ankle bone and Achilles
 tendon on the little toe side.

AROMATHERAPY
Sandalwood.

HELPFUL HERBS
Cat's claw, **hawthorn**, passionflower.

CAUTION! Women who are pregnant should
not use pressure point Li4.

---

*In spite of the hump, the camel's spine is
straight.*

Bunion

A bunion is formed from an inflamed disc in the great toe. This results in swelling of the inner part of the large joint, possibly causing mild to extreme pain. This condition is thought to be more common in women who wear high heels and tight-fitting shoes.

A new form of surgery called Minimal Incision Surgery is being performed by a few podiatrists. Rather than breaking the joint of the great toe as in traditional surgery, this procedure uses a small incision to grind down the inflamed areas. Operating time is a few hours and recovery time is one to six weeks.

Gently massage the area with an aloe vera cream or gel to help reduce inflammation and soreness.

Bunion

TOPICAL TREATMENT
Apply aloe vera gel to the inflamed joint.

LIFE PATTERNS
Take off your shoes. Try walking in bare feet when possible.

MASSAGE
Gently massage the bunion and surrounding area several times daily.

HELPFUL HERBS
Aloe Vera juice, **lemon balm**, parsley tea.

TIP! Gout is a condition of arthritis caused by a build-up of uric acid in the body. It frequently attacks the joint of the great toe and is often thought to be a bunion. Gout attacks mostly occur at night, and usually follow evenings of alcoholic consumption and rich foods that help produce uric acid. Gout is a condition that affects mostly men over the age of thirty.

A homeopathic remedy, arnica ointment or gel, is a favorite home treatment. Arnica ointment or gel can be gently massaged into the feet for reducing swelling, soreness and joint pain. This remedy can be purchased at major health food stores.

Bursitis

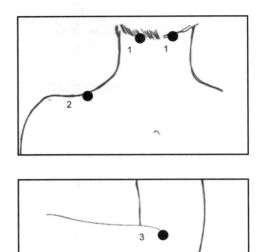

The bursa is a sac-like structure, filled with synovial fluid, that cushions areas that experience friction. This is usually an area that requires mobility and frequent movement. Most people associate bursitis with the shoulder, but there are other joints in the body with bursas, such as the hips and joints in the hands. This condition is almost always painful.

Bursitis

PRESSURE POINTS
1. **Gb20*** At the base of the skull one inch
        either side of the spine.

2. **Gb21** Half way between the neck and
        shoulder joint.

3. **Li11*** At the end of the elbow crease.

TOPICAL TREATMENT
Moist heat. Place moist warm towels over the
inflamed area for twenty minutes. Massage
aloe vera, **comfrey**, or **lemon balm** over the
sore muscles and soft tissue.

HELPFUL HERBS
Chamomile tea, **St. John's wort**.

CAUTION! Women who are pregnant should
not use pressure point Gb21.

Carpal Tunnel Syndrome

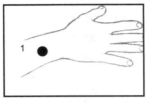 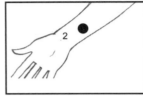

A person may experience numbness, tingling, weakness, or pain in the hand, forearm, or arm, due to a pinch of the median nerve that exits from the sixth cervical vertebra. If you want to locate the sixth vertebra, tilt your head forward and feel the back of your neck. About four inches below the hairline is a large bump, the seventh cervical vertebra. The sixth vertebra is just above it.

    More commonly, the numbness, weakness, and tingling of the hand and fingers is caused by the pinching of the median nerve at the wrist. The carpal bones and surrounding soft tissue expand and pinch the median nerve as it crosses the wrist.

    The easiest technique for massaging these two points is placing the pad of the index or middle finger on TW5 and the pad of the thumb on Pc6. Begin with a gentle massaging motion and activate both points at the same time. Massage for up to one minute and repeat the procedure on the other arm.

Carpal Tunnel Syndrome

PRESSURE POINTS
1. **TW5** Two inches above the wrist on the
   back of the arm.

2. **Pc6** Two inches above the wrist on the
   palm side of the arm.

TOPICAL TREATMENT
Apply a cold compress or ice wrapped in a
towel on the palm side of the wrist.

HELPFUL HERBS
EXTERNAL - cayenne, **comfrey**, wintergreen.
INTERNAL - astwaganda, **St. John's wort**.

Repetitive Motion Syndrome is commonly
known as Carpal Tunnel Syndrome.

*Anyone who performs the same movement
over a period of time will have some
discomfort. One client, a blackjack dealer,
was experiencing low back pain from standing
in one position at the casino table too long.
She now has less discomfort because of the
following therapy tip: she places one foot on a
three-inch wooden block while dealing cards.
This position tilts the pelvis forward and
relaxes the low back muscles. Nurses have
used this technique for many years while
working bedside with patients.*

Chronic Fatigue

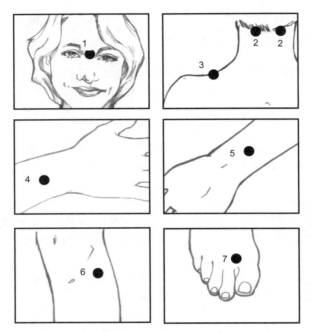

Also referred to as Epstein-Barr Syndrome, this chronic condition can interfere with work performance, socialization, and relationships. Believed to be a viral infection, symptoms can be headaches, irritability, lethargy, and depression.

CAUTION! Women who are pregnant should not use pressure point Gb21.

Chronic Fatigue

PRESSURE POINTS

1. Yin Tang On the bridge of the nose
between the eyebrows. PRESS ONLY

2. Gb20* At the base of the skull one inch
either side of the spine.

3. Gb21 Half way between the neck and
shoulder joint.

4. TW5 Two inches above the center of the
wrist on the back side of the arm.

5. Pc6 Two inches above the center of the
wrist on the palm side.

6. St36* Three inches below the knee next to
the shin bone.

7. Lv3* One inch above the web of the great
and second toe.

AROMATHERAPY
Ginger, peppermint.

HELPFUL HERBS
Cocoa, coffee, **ginger**, ginseng,
St. John's wort.

CAUTION! Women who are pregnant should
not use pressure point Gb21.

Constipation

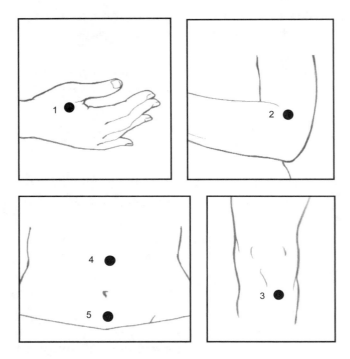

Constipation is a condition that can be caused from a poor diet, poor bowel habits, or problems in elimination of stool, whether physical, functional, or voluntary. Many pharmaceutical products can cause constipation: antacids containing aluminum hydroxide and calcium carbonate, antispasmodic drugs, antidepressants, iron tablets, anticonvulsant drugs, and narcotic-containing drugs.

Constipation

PRESSURE POINTS
1. Li4* Web of the hand.

2. Li11* Edge of the crease in the elbow.

3. St36* Three inches below the knee next to the shin bone.

4. CV12 Three inches above the navel.
PRESS ONLY

5. CV6 One and one-half inches below the navel. PRESS ONLY

AROMATHERAPY
Geranium, lavender.

HELPFUL HERBS
Chamomile, **ginger**, milk thistle.

Note that many of the points for treating con-stipation are also used for treating diar-rhea. These pressure points help to return bodily functions to normalcy.

CAUTION! Women who are pregnant should not use pressure point Li4.
IMPORTANT! Press abdominal points with *gentle pressure.*

Cough

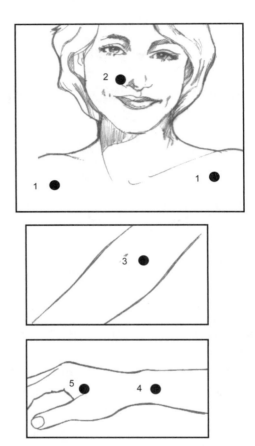

Although a cough is usually initiated by the "automatic" cough reflex, it is a defense against smoke, mis-swallowed food, nasal mucus, and other elements that might accidentally enter the airway. Asthma can also cause coughing due to inflammation of the airway.

Cough

PRESSURE POINTS
1. Lu1 In the shoulder depression two inches
below the collar bone.

2. Li20 On the lateral crease of the nose.
PRESS ONLY

3. Lu5 At the middle of the bend in the elbow.

4. Lu7 Two inches from the wrist on the
thumb side in the small depression.

5. Li4* Web of the hand.

AROMATHERAPY
Eucalyptus, sage.

HELPFUL HERBS
Cat's claw, **chamomile**, **cinnamon**, **comfrey**,
ginger, peppermint.

CAUTION! Women who are pregnant should
not use pressure point Li4.

---

*When you sneeze, your uvula and the soft
pallet of the back of your throat automatically
block your mouth, and all that air is funneled
through small nasal passages. Fastest
laboratory-tested sneeze is 130 mph. The
average cough is between 60 to 70 mph.*

Depression

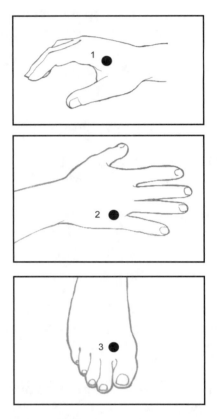

A depressive disorder is an illness that involves the body, mood, and mental state. It affects the lifestyle, the way a person eats and sleeps, one's self-esteem, and the way one perceives people and events. Symptoms can be persistent sadness, anxiety, hopelessness, guilt, appetite changes, weight loss, insomnia, or over-sleeping.

Depression

PRESSURE POINTS
1. **Li4*** Web of the hand.

2.**TW3** On the back of the hand one inch from the web of the little and fourth finger.

3. **Lv3*** About one inch above the web between the great and second toe.

AROMATHERAPY
Orange blossom, strawberry.

HELPFUL HERBS
Ginkgo, **kava, lemon balm, St. John's wort**.

CAUTION! Women who are pregnant should not use pressure point Li4.

The expression of "being under the weather" comes from the idea that bad weather might affect a person's health and mood. The saying also may be related to "under the weather bow," the part of a boat that will take the force of rough seas during stormy weather. If you were in that part of the boat, you might suffer from seasickness.

Diarrhea

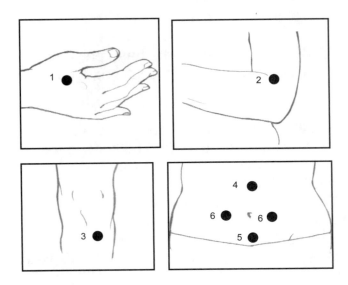

Viral infections, which cause most cases of diarrhea, typically bring mild to moderate symptoms with frequent, watery bowel movements, abdominal cramps, and low-grade fevers. Diarrhea generally lasts from three to seven days.

Bacterial infections cause the more serious cases of diarrhea. You typically get bacteria from contaminated foods or drinks (food poisoning). Bacterial infections can cause severe symptoms with vomiting, fever, and severe abdominal cramps or abdominal pain.

Diarrhea

PRESSURE POINTS
1. Li4* Web of the hand.

2. Li11* Edge of the crease in the elbow.

3. St36* Three inches below the knee next to the shin bone.

4. CV12 Three inches above the navel.
PRESS ONLY

5. CV6 One and one-half inches below the navel. PRESS ONLY

6. St25 About two inches either side of the navel. PRESS ONLY

AROMATHERAPY
Apple, geranium.

HELPFUL HERBS
Bilberry, **lemon balm**, **yarrow**.

CAUTION! Women who are pregnant should not use pressure point Li4.
IMPORTANT! Press abdominal points with gentle pressure.

Dizziness

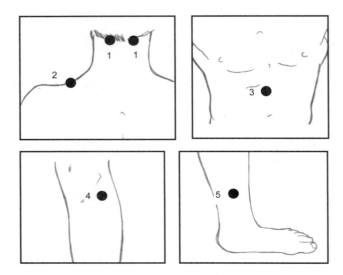

Dizziness, also referred to as vertigo, often originates in the semicircular canals of the middle ear. This is usually due to the head experiencing unusual or sudden motion and sometimes is accompanied by nausea. The above pressure points and the herb ginger are effective in reducing or eliminating dizziness.

IMPORTANT! This condition can be a symptom of more serious medical problems. If dizziness or other related symptoms continue, medical assistance should be sought immediately.

Dizziness

1. **Gb20*** At the base of the skull one inch either side of the spine.

2. **Gb21** Midway between the neck and outer shoulder on the top edge.

3. **CV12** Three inches above the navel.
   PRESS ONLY

4. **St36*** Three inches below the knee next to the shin bone.

5. **Sp6*** Three inches above the inside ankle bone.

AROMATHERAPY
Ginger, peppermint.

HELPFUL HERBS
Cinnamon, **ginger**, ginkgo.

CAUTION! Women who are pregnant should not use pressure points Gb21 and Sp6.

Falls from dizziness causes nearly 100,000 injuries each year. Decrease dizziness by standing slowly and keeping your gaze straight ahead, avoid sudden changes in head position, such as quickly looking up, and use hand rails and walking devices for stability.

Earache

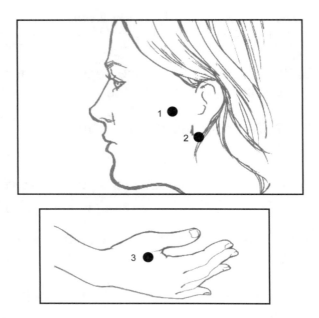

Pain in the ear can occur because of irritation within the ear, the ear canal, or the visible portion of the ear called the Pinna. Acute middle ear infection, medically called acute otitis(ear inflammation) media, and is the most frequent diagnosis in sick children in the United States. The eustachian tube in children allows easy entry of bacteria and viruses into the middle ear. This results in middle ear inflammation. Infection of the ear canal (otitis externa) is also called swimmer's ear.

Earache

PRESSURE POINTS
1. **St19** About one inch in front of the ear, should be massaged with the mouth open.

2. **TW17** In the depression behind the ear lobe. PRESS ONLY

3. **Li4*** In the web of the hand.

AROMATHERAPY
Lavender.

HELPFUL HERBS
Chamomile, lavender, lemon balm.

CAUTION! Women who are pregnant should not use pressure point Li4.

The gentle heat from a hair dryer may help alleviate the pain of an earache. The heat of the hair dryer will melt the earwax which serves as a protective coating over the exposed eardrum.

Eye Strain

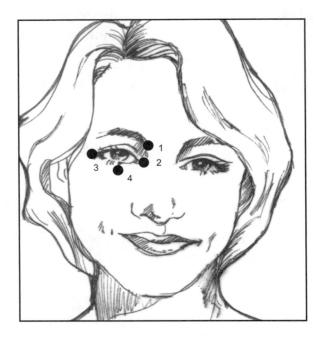

Eye strain often occurs from overuse of the eye muscles. Any muscle held in one position for long periods of time will cause fatigue and strain. When concentrating on a task such as reading, working at the computer or watching television for any length of time, the inner eye muscles tighten causing the eyes to become irritated, dry and uncomfortable. Giving the eyes a chance to refocus once or twice an hour for five minutes reduces the strain. A cool moist compress for one minute can also help refresh the eyes.

Eye Strain

PRESSURE POINTS
For maximum benefit, press right and left
points for each location at the same time using
fingers or thumbs.
1. **B2** Inside corner of the eyebrows.
   PRESS ONLY

2. **B1** Next to the inside corner of the eye.
   PRESS ONLY

3. **Gb1** Next to the outside corner of the eye.
   PRESS ONLY

4. **St1** On the edge of the bone of the lower
   eye socket. PRESS ONLY

AROMATHERAPY
Lavender, lemon balm, linden blossom,
orange blossom.

HELPFUL HERBS
Cool water compress with a few drops of
linden blossom, **lavender**, or **lemon balm**
added to the water.

CAUTION! Proper hygiene is important to
prevent infections of the eye and the
conjunctiva around the eye.

Most people blink about 17,000 times a day.

Fatigue, Tiredness

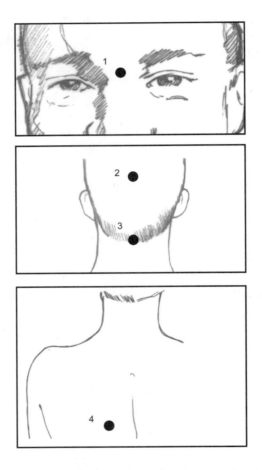

Fatigue and tiredness are natural ways the body is asking for rest and relaxation to re-energize. Products, such as stimulants, have a short-term effect and will actually increase the fatigue.

Fatigue, Tiredness

PRESSURE POINTS
1. Yin Tang On the bridge of the nose between the eyes. PRESS ONLY

2. GV19 On the posterior fontanel at the back of the head. PRESS ONLY

3. GV16 Midline in the hollow of the base of the skull.

4. Gb24 Next to the scapula between the fifth and sixth rib.

AROMATHERAPY
Peppermint, strawberry.

HELPFUL HERBS
Chamomile, cocoa, coffee, **kava, St. John's wort**.

Homeostasis is the body's natural defense to maintain a balance or equilibrium of function. Ingesting foods, such as chocolate or sugar, naturally triggers the pancreas to release insulin, since the insulin is necessary to help metabolize the sugar. This is the Citric Acid Cycle, which brings the blood sugar down to the previous level. The problems begin when the pancreas malfunctions with too much or too little insulin, hence the terms "hyperglycemia" and "hypoglycemia."

Fever

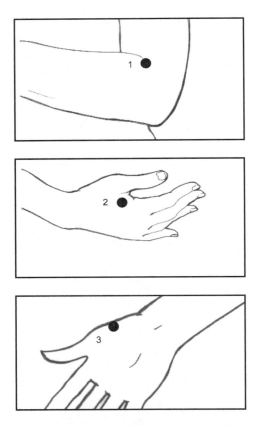

A fever is not an illness but can be a defense against infection. Because bacteria and viruses are comfortable at the body's normal temperature, 98.6 F. or 35 C., increasing the temperature by a few degrees can stop the growth and spread of bacteria and viruses.

Fever

PRESSURE POINTS
1. **Li11*** Corner of the crease in the elbow.

2. **Li4*** Web of the hand.

3. **Lu10** Midpoint between the wrist and first joint of the thumb.

AROMATHERAPY
Lavender.

HELPFUL HERBS
Cinnamon, lavender.

CAUTION! Women who are pregnant should not use pressure point Li4.

A lukewarm bath or sponge bath may help cool someone with a fever. Using cold baths or alcohol rubs cool the skin, but often make the situation worse by causing shivering, which raises the core body temperature.

Hay fever is not a fever, but an allergic reaction to pollen from grasses, blooms, trees, and weeds. Conditions from hay fever usually increase in spring or onset of warm weather.

Hangover

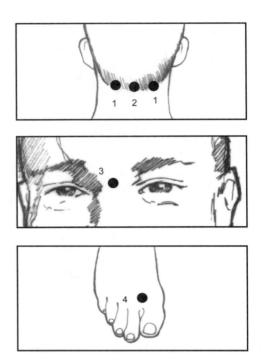

If you have ever suffered from this malady, you know how uncomfortable it can be. The primary cause is the over-ingestion of alcoholic beverages the previous night. Together with the headache and general sluggish feeling is the impaired sensory processing and decreased cognition.

Hangover

PRESSURE POINTS

1. Gb20* The base of the skull one inch
either side of the spine.

2. GV16 Midline at the base of the skull.

3. Yin Tang The bridge of the nose between
the eyebrows. PRESS ONLY

4. Lv3* One inch above the web of the great
and second toe.

SELF-CARE TREATMENT
HYDROTHERAPY
Take a hot shower or spray followed by a
cold rinse. A steam bath or sauna can be
helpful, but fluid intake is essential. Drink a lot
of non-alcoholic fluids because alcohol
dehydrates the body.

HELPFUL HERBS
TREATMENT - **ginger**, ginseng, **lavender**, **St.
John's wort**, soy lecithin, willow bark.
PREVENTION - aloe, Chinese senega root.

*The human body is able to metabolize about
one-half oz. of alcohol each hour and is
absorbed directly into the blood stream
through tissue lining the stomach and small
intestine. Food, water, and fruit juice help to
slow this absorption, while carbonation tends
to speed absorption.*

Headaches

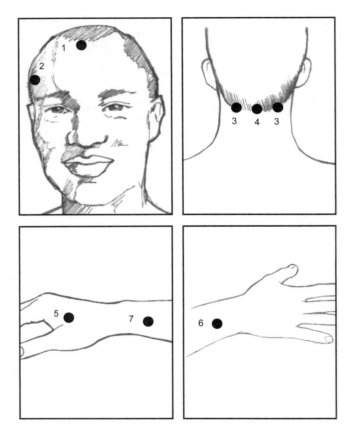

Headaches, one of the most common
ailments, affects thousands of Americans
every day. The symptoms and pain associated
with the various types of headache can be
difficult to identify. This makes it hard to pin
point the exact type of headache and the best
treatment for it.

Headaches

PRESSURE POINTS

1. GV23 Midline at the hairline. PRESS ONLY

2. Gb13 Over the outside corner of the eye at the hairline. PRESS ONLY

3. Gb20* At the base of the skull one inch on either side of the spine.

4. GV16 In the depression at the base of the skull.

5. Li4* Web of the hand.

6. TW5 Two inches above the wrist on the back of the arm.

7. Lu7 Two inches above the wrist in the small depression on the thumb side.

AROMATHERAPY
Orange blossom.

HELPFUL HERBS
Cayenne, **chamomile**, **lavender**.

CAUTION! Women who are pregnant should not use pressure point Li4.

Hemorrhoids

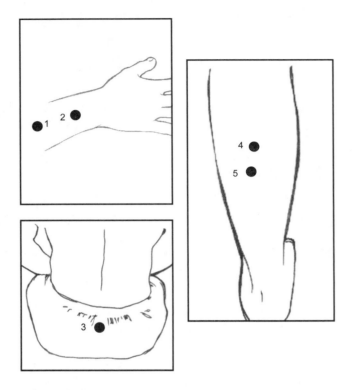

Hemorrhoids, also known as varicose veins, are a condition in which the veins around the anus, or in the anal canal, become swollen when stretched under pressure. Hemorrhoids are probably the most common cause of visible blood in the digestive tract, especially blood that appears bright red. They are not dangerous, although they can be very annoying and painful.

Hemorrhoids

PRESSURE POINTS
1. **Li6** On the back of the arm midway between the wrist and elbow.

2. **TW5** Two inches above the wrist on the back of the arm.

3. **GV2** At the fold of the buttocks between the sacrum and coccyx.

4. **B57** At the V-shape of the calf muscle on the back of the leg.

5. **B58** One inch below and to the outside of B57.

AROMATHERAPY
Chamomile.

HELPFUL HERBS
EXTERNAL: aloe, **St. John's Wort**, witch hazel.
INTERNAL: butcher's broom, **chamomile**, dandelion.

There are 60,000 miles (97,000 km) of blood vessels in every human.

Hiccups

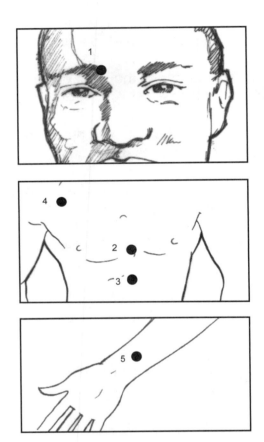

A hiccup is a spasm of the diaphragm. When the diaphragm becomes irritated, it pushes up in a jerking movement that makes the breath come out differently from a normal pattern. When this irregular breath hits the voice box, the result is a big hiccup.

Hiccups

PRESSURE POINTS

1. B2 At the corner of the eyebrow near the bridge of the nose. PRESS ONLY

2. CV17 Midpoint at the center of the sternum.

3. CV12 Midline of the body about two inches below the sternum.

4. Lu1 In the shoulder depression two inches below the collar bone.

5. Pc6 Two inches above the crease of the wrist on the palm side of the forearm.

AROMATHERAPY
Clove.

HELPFUL HERBS
Cinnamon, **comfrey**, **ginger**.

Some old wives tales for ridding hiccups:
Holding your breath as long as possible.
Drinking a large glass of ice water will help at least to calm down the hiccups.
Breathe deeply and slowly, holding air in long enough to let the lungs convey oxygen into your bloodstream.
Swallow a spoon of sugar or let a sugar cube dissolve in the mouth before swallowing.

High Blood Pressure

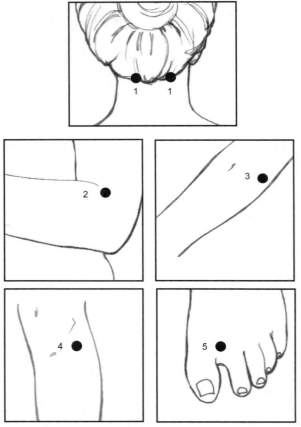

Nearly one in three U.S. adults has high blood pressure, and nearly one-third of these people don't know they have it. This condition can lead to stroke, heart attack, heart or kidney failure. High blood pressure is often called the "silent killer."

High Blood Pressure

PRESSURE POINTS
1. **Gb20*** Just below the base of the skull, one inch on either side of the spine.

2. **Li11*** Edge of the elbow crease.

3. **Ht3** One inch above the crease of the elbow on the little finger side.

4. **St36*** Three inches below the knee cap and just to the outside edge of the shin bone.

5. **Lv3*** About one inch above the web of the great and second toes.

AROMATHERAPY
Orange blossom.

HELPFUL HERBS
American ginseng, bilberry, coleus, ginseng, **hawthorn**.

CAUTION! This condition may be a warning of more serious conditions and should not be taken lightly. Medical assistance should be sought immediately.

Indigestion

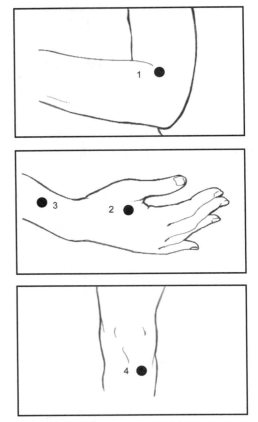

Indigestion can result from over-eating, from consuming spicy foods or alcoholic beverages. Also referred to as "heartburn," indigestion can be related to more serious conditions, such as ulcers and diverticulitis. If indigestion persists for more than two days, seek medical attention.

Indigestion

PRESSURE POINTS
1. **Li11*** On the outside crease of the elbow.

2. **Li4*** Web of the hand.

3. **Lu7** Two inches from the wrist on the thumb side in the small depression.

4. **St36*** Three inches below the knee next to the shin bone.

AROMATHERAPY
Peppermint.

HELPFUL HERBS
Cat's claw, **cinnamon**, **comfrey**, fennel seed, **ginger**, **lemon balm**, peppermint.

CAUTION! Women who are pregnant should not use pressure point Li4.

Allow time for leisurely meals. Chew food carefully and thoroughly. Avoid conflicts during meals. Avoid excitement or exercise immediately after a meal. Avoid chewing gum; it may cause air swallowing. A calm environment and rest may help relieve stress-related dyspepsia.

Insomnia

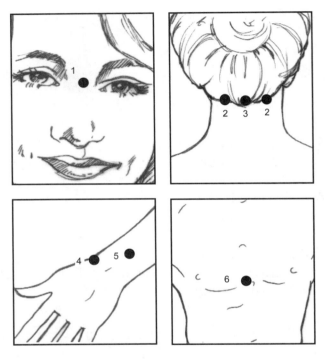

People with this sleep disorder called insomnia have one or more of the following symptoms: difficulty falling asleep, waking up often during the night and having trouble going back to sleep, waking up too early in the morning, or unrefreshing sleep. Other serious sleep disorders are sleep apnea, not breathing during sleep for 10 seconds or more; narcolepsy, periodically falling asleep during the day; and restless leg syndrome, shaking movements of the leg preventing sleep.

Insomnia

PRESSURE POINTS
1. **Yin Tang** On the bridge of the nose
   between the eyebrows. PRESS ONLY

2. **Gb20*** Just below the base of the skull one
   inch on either side of the spine.

3. **GV16** Midline at the base of the skull.

4. **Ht7** On the wrist crease in line with the little
   finger.

5. **Pc6** Two inches above the center of the
   wrist on the palm side.

6. **CV17** Midpoint at the center of the sternum.
   PRESS ONLY

AROMATHERAPY
Lavender, rosemary.

HELPFUL HERBS
Chamomile, **kava**, **lavender**, **lemon balm**,
passionflower, **St. John's wort**, **yarrow**.

*The average person falls asleep in seven
minutes. Recent research suggests that
people who sleep four hours or less each
night may have a higher risk for weight gain
than people who sleep at least seven hours
each night.*

Jet Lag

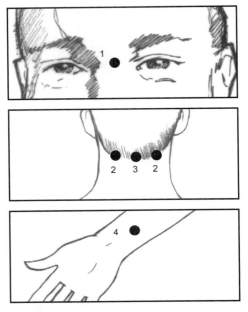

Whether traveling across several time zones or half way around the world, distant traveling upsets our "biological clock" which tells us when to eat, when to wake up, and when to sleep. Because our physical, mental, and even spiritual well-being are off center; we are likely to experience sluggishness and lethargy. To combat this syndrome, make some simple adjustments. Before the flight, eat a meal high in protein, such as eggs, meat, fish, or cheese; skip the Danish. For supper, eat a modest meal of protein, carbohydrates, and fats, but skip the chocolate eclair.

Jet Lag

PRESSURE POINTS
1. Yin Tang Bridge of the nose between the
eye brows. PRESS ONLY

2. Gb20* On the base of the skull one inch
either side of the spine.

3. GV16 Midline at the base of the skull.

4. Pc6 Two inches from the wrist in the center
of the palm side of the forearm.

PHYSICAL ACTIVITY
Move around. Movement promotes circulation.
Elevate your feet if possible to prevent
swelling.
Go for a brisk walk after the flight to increase
circulation and oxygenation.

MASSAGE
Massage the hands and feet every two hours
to reduce swelling during the flight.

AROMATHERAPY
Eucalyptus, peppermint, strawberry.

HELPFUL HERBS
Cinnamon, cocoa, coffee, **ginger**, ginseng,
kava, kola.

Joint Pain

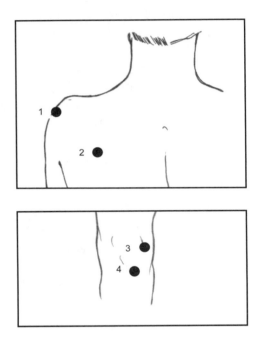

Joint pain can be caused by many types of injuries or conditions. No matter what causes it, joint pain can be very intense. Common causes can be unusual exertion or overuse, including strains or sprains; injury including fracture, gout (commonly found in the big toe), osteoarthritis; infectious diseases, such as septic arthritis, tendonitis, bursitis, measles (rubeola and rubella), mumps, Epstein-Barr syndrome, and autoimmune diseases; such as lupus and rheumatoid arthritis.

Joint Pain

PRESSURE POINTS
1. Li15 On the outer edge of the shoulder.

2. Si11 On the center of the scapula.

3. St35 Outer side of the knee joint.

4. St36* Three inches below the knee cap
and just to the outside of the shin bone.

AROMATHERAPY
Eucalyptus, juniper.

HELPFUL HERBS
Alfalfa, **cat's claw**, cayenne, **ginger.
hawthorn**, willow bark, yucca.

*Joint pain can interfere with two measurable
functions of joint movement; range of motion
and strength. A warm moist towel applied to a
painful joint can bring relief by promoting
circulation. Massaging the skin with a warmed
oil can also promote circulation and provide
temporary relief.*
*The oil is as important as the massage.
Synthetic oils, such as petroleum and mineral
oil, coat the skin and clog the pores.
Vegetable oil is closer to the skin's natural oil,
unfortunately, many of these oils contain
synthetics. Select an organic natural oil for
massage and skin application.*

Laryngitis

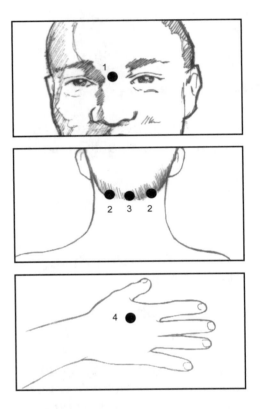

This is an inflammation of the larynx, located at the base of the throat, causing a raspy voice, scratchy feeling, discomfort and pain. Causes can be from yelling and screaming, bacterial and viral infection, and allergies.

Laryngitis

PRESSURE POINTS

1. **Yin Tang** Between the eye brows at the bridge of the nose.

2. **Gb20*** One inch either side of the midline of the skull.

3. **GV16** Midline at the base of the skull.

4. **Li4*** Web of the hand.

TOPICAL TREATMENT
Apply a cold compress to the throat.

CAUTION! Women who are pregnant should not use pressure point Li4.

AROMATHERAPY
Frankincense, lavender, sandalwood.

HELPFUL HERBS
A warm gargle (do not swallow) with bayberry, **chamomile**, cranesbill, or sage tea.

Laryngitis can also be caused by inhaling irritants, such as smoke, chemicals, dust and toxic fumes. You may have noticed that more painters, carpenters, farm workers, and others are wearing respirators and dust masks to protect the lungs and throat.

Leg Cramps

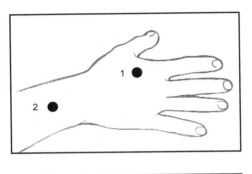

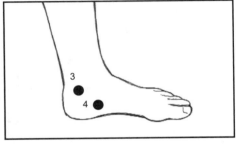

Leg cramps refers to a painful, involuntary contraction of a single muscle or a muscle group. Leg cramps frequently occur in the legs of elderly, bedridden patients and can be extremely painful. Severe leg cramps may be followed by residual tenderness and evidence of muscle fiber deterioration. Complaints of muscle pain and muscle fatigue are among the most frequent symptoms. Such pain and fatigue can be particularly troublesome during pregnancy

Leg Cramps

PRESSURE POINTS

1. Li4* Web of the hand.

2. TW5 Two inches above the wrist on the back of the forearm.

3. Kd3* Point between the inside ankle bone and Achilles tendon.

4. Kd2 One inch below the inside ankle bone.

AROMATHERAPY
Rosemary.

HELPFUL HERBS
Chamomile, ginger, yarrow.

CAUTION! Women who are pregnant should not use pressure point Li4.

When legs begin to cramp, stretch the legs. Athletes learned that stretching before a sporting event reduced muscle cramping If the calf muscle cramps, straighten the knee. Reach down, grab the ball of the foot, and pull toward you. Stretching the muscle helps reduce the cramping. Hold this position until the muscles relax.

Low Blood Pressure

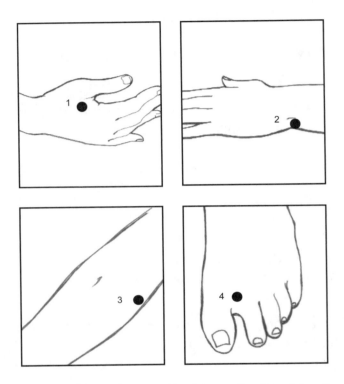

Hypotension is the medical term for low blood pressure (below 90/60). Low blood pressure that does not cause symptoms is generally considered to be a sign of good cardiovascular health because there is less stress on the heart and blood vessels. People should seek treatment for low blood pressure if they experience symptoms such as dizziness or fainting from lack of oxygen to the brain.

Low Blood Pressure

PRESSURE POINTS

1. Li4* Web of the hand.

2. Ht7 At the crease of the wrist on the little finger side.

3. Ht3 One inch above the elbow bone on the little finger side.

4. Lv3* About one inch above the web of the great and second toes.

AROMATHERAPY
Rosemary.

HELPFUL HERBS
Coltsfoot, licorice.

> CAUTION! Women who are pregnant should not use pressure point Li4.

One cause of low blood pressure is anaphylaxis, a severe allergic reaction, that affects the entire body. After an initial exposure to a substance, such as a bee sting, the immune system becomes sensitized to that allergen. On a subsequent exposure, an allergic reaction occurs. This reaction is sudden, severe, and involves the entire body.

Memory and Cognition Problems

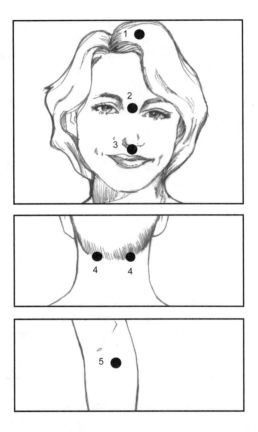

Poor mental function, difficulty remembering, and difficulty in focusing and following information are typical memory and cognition problems. Possible causes are Alzheimer's, allergies, low blood sugar, infection, amino acid imbalance, and stroke.

Memory and Cognition Problems

PRESSURE POINTS

1. GV20 Midline at the top of the head.
PRESS ONLY

2. Yin Tang Midline between the eye brows.
PRESS ONLY

3. GV26 Midline between the nose and upper lip. PRESS ONLY

4. Gb20* One inch either side of the spine at the base of the skull.

5. St36* Three inches below the knee cap and just to the outside of the shin bone.

VISUAL-PERCEPTUAL THERAPY
This type of therapy may be effective for improving mental focus. Therapies are conducted to improve visual and mental focus on a variety of topics. After several sessions of practicing techniques, the individual is asked to recall learned information by oral or written communication.

AROMATHERAPY
Peppermint, strawberry, tangerine.

HELPFUL HERBS
Ginkgo leaf extract, ginseng.

Menstrual Cramps

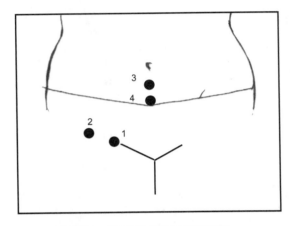

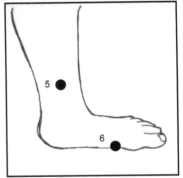

Menstrual cramps start a day or so before
actual menses and are felt in the lower or
middle abdomen. They can radiate to the hips,
thighs, and back. The pain the produce rises
to a peak and falls, then starts over again due
to the contractions of the uterus that underlie
the cramps.

Menstrual Cramps

PRESSURE POINTS

1. Sp12 Midway on the leg crease at the pelvis. PRESS ONLY

2. Sp13 One-half inch above Sp12 on the leg crease. PRESS ONLY

3. CV6 About two inches below the navel. PRESS ONLY

4. CV4 About three inches below the navel. PRESS ONLY

5. Sp6* Three inches above the inside ankle bone.

6. Sp4 On the arch of the foot, one inch from the great toe.

AROMATHERAPY
Lavender, rosemary

HELPFUL HERBS
Chamomile, **cinnamon**, Dong quai, **ginger**, shepherd's purse, **yarrow**.

Body temperature varies less in adults than children. However, a woman's menstrual cycle can elevate her temperature by one degree or more.

Migraines

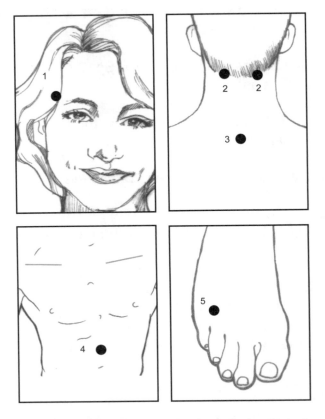

Migraines, vascular headaches thought to be caused by abnormal function of the circulatory system, affect one in eight adults in the developed world. People of any age can suffer, although adults aged 25 to 34 are most commonly affected, and women two or three times as frequently as men.

Migraines

PRESSURE POINTS

1. Tai Yang In the depression one inch from the outer corner of the eye. PRESS ONLY

2. Gb20* The base of the skull one inch either side of the spine.

3. GV12 Located on the third thoracic vertebra. Tilting the head forward, locate the bump about four inches below the base of the skull; this is C7. Three inches below this point is GV12.

4. CV12 Three inches above the navel.
PRESS ONLY

5. Gb41 On top of the foot between the fourth and little toe.

AROMATHERAPY
Marjoram.

HELPFUL HERBS
Cayenne, ginkgo, **St. John's wort**, tilden flower.

Tension, bright lights, loud noises, strong smells, weather changes, fatigue, missed meals, and emotional upset may trigger a migraine, as well as artificial sweeteners, nuts, cheeses, coffee, teas, and chocolate.

Muscular Cramps

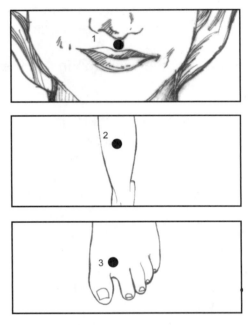

Skeletal muscles have a natural amount of contraction called *muscle tone*. When excessive or abnormal tone in the muscles occurs they may produce spasms, cramps, and twitches can be the symptoms. Other symptoms are discomfort, tightness, tingling, and burning. Although these conditions are not uncommon to most people once in a while, they are most common in those who are sedentary, lack regular exercise, have low levels of magnesium, or on a diet that reduces calcium in the body.

Muscular Cramps

PRESSURE POINTS
1. GV26 Midline between the nose and
upper lip. PRESS ONLY

2. B57 At the V-shape of the calf muscle
on the back of the leg.

3. Lv3* One inch above the web of the great
and second toes.

TOPICAL TREATMENT
Apply a warm compress to affected area as
needed. Leave on for ten minutes and off ten
minutes. Repeat procedure for up to one hour.

AROMATHERAPY
Chamomile, lavender, marjoram, rosemary.

HELPFUL HERBS
Chamomile, cramp bark tea, **lavender**.

*In addition to the stretching exercise for
stopping leg cramps, warmth also has a
positive effect in reducing cramps. Wearing
clothing that provides comfort and warmth will
help prevent cramping, and covering the legs
and ankles during activities will reduce leg
cramping.*

Nausea

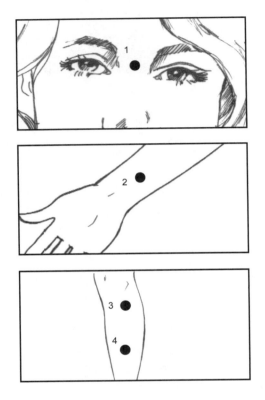

Nausea and vomiting are not diseases, but symptoms of many different conditions, such as stomach flu, food poisoning, motion sickness, over-eating, blocked intestine, illness, concussion or brain injury, appendicitis and migraines. Nausea is an uneasiness of the stomach that often accompanies the urge to vomit, but doesn't always lead to vomiting.

Nausea

PRESSURE POINTS

1. Yin Tang On the bridge of the nose
between the eyebrows. PRESS ONLY

2. Pc6 Two inches above the wrist in the
center of the arm on the palm side.

3. St36* Three inches below the knee cap
beside the edge of the shin bone.

4. St40* Middle of the lower leg two inches to
the outside of the shin bone.

AROMATHERAPY
Ginger, peppermint.

HELPFUL HERBS
**Cinnamon, comfrey, ginger, lavender,
lemon balm**, peppermint, **St. John's wort**.

*Ginger can help settle upset stomachs and
ease nausea. Studies have shown that ginger
may be up to three times more effective at
stopping motion sickness than the common
over-the-counter medication. Ginger is also
the most frequently used herb in the world.*

Neck and Shoulder Tension

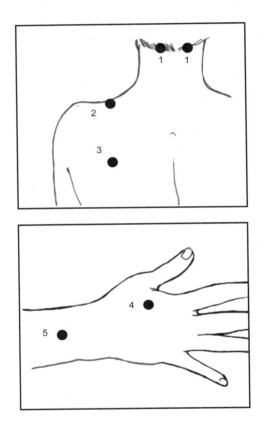

Neck and shoulder tension can result in headaches, back pain, nausea, even migraines. Reducing this tension can help to rid some of these chronic problems. In addition to the pressure points, a warm shower or bath and a five-minute gentle massage can reduce this condition.

Neck and Shoulder Tension

PRESSURE POINTS
1. **Gb20*** At the base of the skull one inch to either side of the spine.

2. **Gb21** On the ridge between the neck and shoulder.

3. **Si11** The center of the scapula.

4. **Li4*** Web of the hand.

5. **TW5** Two inches from the wrist on the back of the forearm.

AROMATHERAPY
Lavender.

HELPFUL HERBS
Chamomile, **kava**, **lavender**, passionflower.

CAUTION! Women who are pregnant should not use pressure points Li4 and Gb21.

The neck supports the weight of the head and is the conduit for the nervous system and an intricate network of muscles and vessels. The human head contributes about 8% to the total body weight, so if your weight is 150 lbs., your head weighs about twelve pounds.

Neuralgia, Neuritis

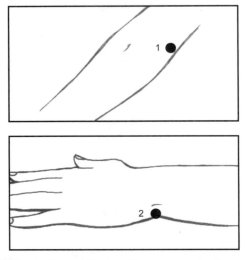

Neuralgia and neuritis occur in the peripheral nervous system, those nerves outside of the spinal cord. Simply stated, neuralgia is the inflammation of the nerve, and the inflamed nerve causes the pain and discomfort. Neuritis is the inflammation of the tissue around the nerve. The inflamed tissue, pressing on the healthy nerve, causes pain and discomfort. Both of these conditions can be caused by disease, pressure from a spinal disc or pinched nerve, such as carpel tunnel syndrome. Symptoms can be numbness, tingling, burning and acute pain. Although these symptoms are usually short-term when treated, they can lead to chronic discomfort if if left unattended.

Neuralgia, Neuritis

PRESSURE POINTS

1. Ht3 Just above the elbow bone on
the little finger side.

2. Ht7 The indentation just above the
wrist on the little finger side

TOPICAL TREATMENT
Epson Salts compress.

THERMAL TREATMENT
Warm compress for neuralgia conditions.
Cold compress for neuritis conditions.
A warm compress or bath will ease the
discomfort of neuralgia.
A cold compress will shrink inflamed tissue
around the nerve and bring relief to neuritis.

AROMATHERAPY
Eucalyptus, lavender.

HELPFUL HERBS
Cedarwood, juniper, **lavender**, **St. John's
wort**.

Ht3 (1) and Ht7 (2), on the heart meridian,
can help mental well-being and the autonomic
nervous system.

Nose Bleeds

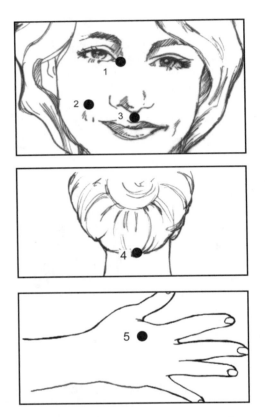

The most common causes are dryness (often caused by indoor heat in the winter) and nose picking. Other, less common causes include injuries, colds, and allergies. You will need to have medical attention if a nosebleed goes on for more than 15 minutes, especially if you have been punched in the nose.

Nose Bleeds

PRESSURE POINTS

1. B1 At the inner corner of the eye.
PRESS ONLY

2. St3 At the bottom of the cheek bone below the eye.

3. GV26 Midline between the upper lip and nose. PRESS ONLY

4. GV16 Midline at the base of the skull.

5. Li4* In the web of the hand between the thumb and index finger.

TOPICAL TREATMENT
If you get a nosebleed, sit down and lean slightly forward. Keeping your head above your heart will make your nose bleed less. A cold compress placed on the bridge of the nose can reduce bleeding.

AROMATHERAPY
Orange blossom.

HELPFUL HERBS
Agrimony, **chamomile**, shepherd's purse, **St. John's wort**, **yarrow**.

CAUTION! Women who are pregnant should not use pressure point Li4.

Pain

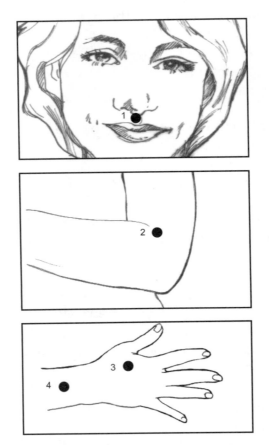

Pain is a word that covers a wide range of sensory and emotional discomforts. The above pressure points are primary points for general pain of the head, abdomen, and upper and lower extremities.

Pain

PRESSURE POINTS

1. GV26 Midline between the upper lip and nose. PRESS ONLY

2. Li11* Edge of the crease of the elbow.

3. Li4* Web of the hand.

4. TW5 Two inches above the wrist on the center of the back forearm.

IMPORTANT!
Care should be expressed when taking medications, prescription or over-the-counter, for pain. Read the enclosed information and talk with a pharmacist or physician about short-term and long-term side effects.

AROMATHERAPY
Chamomile, ginger.

HELPFUL HERBS
Cayenne, **ginger**, **kava**, tumeric, willow bark.

CAUTION! Women who are pregnant should not use pressure point Li4.

Sciatica

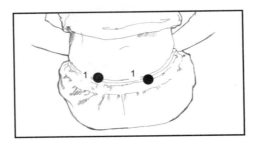

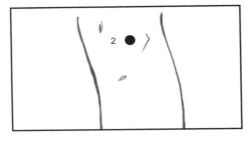

Sciatica can be considered a form of neuralgia or neuritis. Sciatica pain can be extremely intense. It usually begins in the lower back and traveling down the buttocks and thigh. Sometimes the pain may travel down the leg to the foot, following the path of the sciatic nerve. Sciatic neuralgia is usually an inflammation of the nerve, and sciatic neuritis is an irritation of the nerve caused by pinching or pressure from bone, muscle, or trigger point.

Sciatica

PRESSURE POINTS
1. B23* About three inches either side of the
   vertebrae.

2. B54 Back of the knee on the center of the
   crease.

BODY POSITIONING
Lying on the back with knees bent or feet
elevated can bring temporary relief. However,
lying on the stomach can increase irritation
from pinching the sciatic nerve.

THERMAL TREATMENT
A warm compress will help decrease the pain
of neuralgia, but heat will inflame neuritis. For
neuritis use a cold compress to reduce
swelling of surrounding tissue of the nerve.

AROMATHERAPY
Apply a compress of camomile or lavender.

HELPFUL HERBS
Chamomile, **Lavender**, **St. John's Wort**,
Willow bark.

*Exercise is usually better for healing sciatic
pain than bed rest. Bed rest for a day or two
after a sciatica flare-up will help, but after that
time period, inactivity will usually increase the
pain. Walking and moving around are
excellent forms of exercise.*

Sinusitis

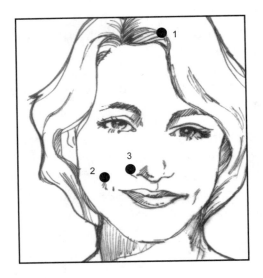

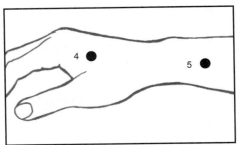

Sinusitis, the inflammation or infection of the paranasal sinuses, occurs when proper drainage of the sinuses is interrupted. This can be an acute condition or chronic, the latter of which may last for several weeks.

Sinusitis

PRESSURE POINTS
1. **GV23** One inch above the hairline directly above the nose.

2. **Si18** Directly down from the eye below the cheekbone.

3. **Li20** The groove next to the nostril.

4. **Li4*** Web of the hand.

5. **Lu7** The thumb-side of the arm two inches above the wrist.

AROMATHERAPY
Eucalyptus.

HELPFUL HERBS
Cat's claw, **chamomile**, **cinnamon**, elderberry, horehound, **St. John's wort**.

CAUTION! Women who are pregnant should not use pressure point Li4.

One reason sinuses do not drain properly is that they may open from the top and not from the bottom. Some people have found temporary relief by lying supine on a bed and tilting the head over the side of the bed to promote draining.

Sore Throat

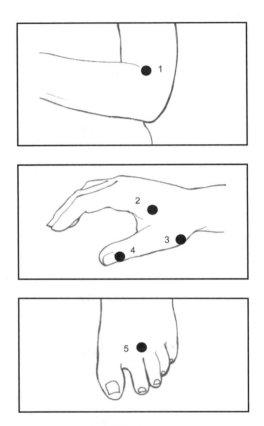

The vast majority of sore throats are caused by viral infections. Many people have a mild sore throat at the beginning of every cold. When the nose or sinuses become infected, drainage can run down the back of the throat and irritate it, especially at night.

Sore Throat

1. **Li11*** Edge of the crease in the elbow.

2. **Li4*** Web of the hand.

3. **Lu10** Between the wrist and first thumb joint on the *palm side* of the hand.

4. **Lu11** Above the nail bed of the thumb.

5. **St44** Top of the foot next to the web of the second and third toes.

AROMATHERAPY
Eucalyptus, peppermint.

HELPFUL HERBS
Comfrey. raspberry leaf tea, **St. John's wort**.

> CAUTION! Women who are pregnant should not use pressure point Li4.

The best ways to avoid catching or passing the viruses and bacteria that can lead to a sore throat are to wash hands regularly, avoid touching the eyes or mouth, and you and others cover the mouth when coughing or sneezing

Sprains

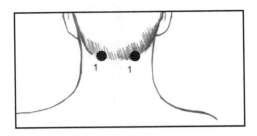

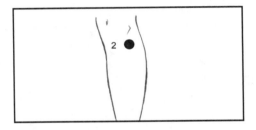

Sprains occur when joints are overstretched or injured, causing damage to the surrounding muscles, connective tissue or even tendons. Sprains can range from mild, with minimal damage and swelling, to severe, with tears in the soft tissue, hemorrhaging under the skin, joint immobility, and muscle spasms. At times a splint may assist in the healing process by protecting the injured tissue from additional damage. This splint may be fabricated from rigid foam material and Velcro closures for easy application and removal.

Sprains

PRESSURE POINTS
1. **Gb20*** One inch either side of the spine at the base of the skull.

2. **St36*** Three inches below the knee cap and just to the outside of the shin bone.

TOPICAL TREATMENT
Apply a cold pack to the affected area twenty minutes each hour for twelve hours.

AROMATHERAPY
Eucalyptus, lavender, wintergreen.

HELPFUL HERBS
Comfrey, horse chestnut, **lavender**, peppermint.

CAUTION!
If swelling continues after applying a cold compress, seek medical attention. This is important especially with sprains of the wrist and ankle. A sprain of the wrist or ankle that does not improve may indicate serious soft tissue damage or bone fracture.

Stress

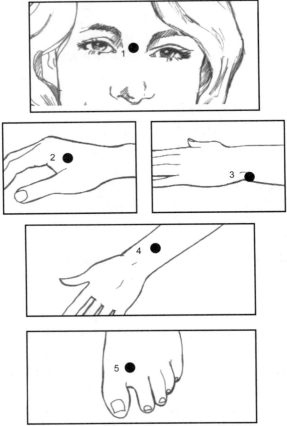

Stress is considered America's number one health problem and is costing this country over $300 billion a year in lost productivity and increased health care costs. Stress is linked to heart attacks, strokes, and depression.

Stress

PRESSURE POINTS

1. Yin Tang On the bridge of the nose
between the eyebrows. PRESS ONLY

2. Li4* Web of the hand.

3. Ht7 The indentation just above the wrist on
the little finger side.

4. Pc6 Two inches above the crease in the
wrist on the palm side.

5. Lv3* One inch above the web of the great
and second toes.

AROMATHERAPY
Lavender, rosemary.

HELPFUL HERBS
Chamomile, **lemon balm**, Siberian ginseng.

CAUTION! Women who are pregnant should not use pressure point Li4.

Tennis Elbow (elbow pain)

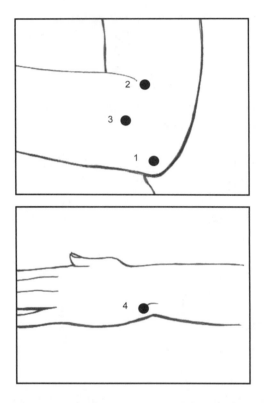

Tennis elbow is a generalized term used for any pain in the elbow region. It has been associated with tennis players who have injured the tendons or bursa of the elbow, but anyone can experience this discomfort through overexertion or even infection.

Tennis Elbow (elbow pain)

PRESSURE POINTS
1. **Si8** Outside of the elbow joint.

2. **Li11*** Outside edge of the crease in the elbow.

3. **Li10** About two inches below the crease of the elbow on the outside.

4. **Si4** The depression just below the wrist on the little finger side.

TOPICAL TREATMENT
Cold pack to inhibit the swelling by applying to the elbow after the injury. After the swelling decreases, apply moist heat to relieve the discomfort. Topical ointments, such as Biofreeze, can also bring temporary relief.

AROMATHERAPY
Chamomile, eucalyptus.

HELPFUL HERBS
Cayenne, **chamomile**, **St. John's wort**, **yarrow**.

Three major nerves travel through the elbow and forearm region. The radial n. lies along the back of the forearm, the median n. is on the palmer side of the forearm, and the ulnar n. is on the little-finger side.

Toothache

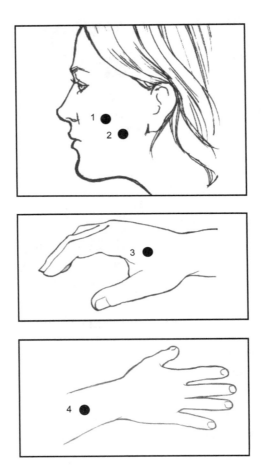

The most common cause of toothache, or pain in the region of the jaws and face, is inflammation of the pulp of the tooth. The short, sharp pains usually occur in response to hot, cold or sweet stimuli.

Toothache

PRESSURE POINTS
1. **St7** Under the cheekbone.

2. **St6** Clench your teeth and locate the muscle at the hinge of the jaw.

3. **Li4*** Web of the hand.

4. **TW5** About two inches above the wrist on the back of the hand.

AROMATHERAPY
Clove

HELPFUL HERBS
Clove, **kava,** thyme, willow bark.

Here are a few tips until you can seek dental help:
Avoid hot, cold or sweet stimuli.
If the pain is caused by exposed root surfaces, toothpaste for sensitive teeth may help.
A saltwater mouthwash can help reduce pain and help heal mouth ulcers.(one tsp. of salt to one cup of warm water.)

CAUTION! Women who are pregnant should not use pressure point Li4.

Helpful Hints and Tips

The following pages contain information for daily use or preventative techniques that make daily activities more comfortable and contribute to general health and wellness. These hints and tips can also be applied for the benefit of friends and family members in need of modified lifestyles for safety and energy conservation.

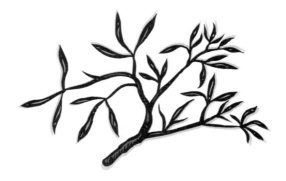

Elastic bandage - ankle injury

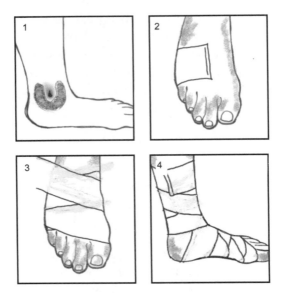

Elastic bandages can be in bright colors of orange, red, purple, green, and generic beige. The bandages can be secured with metal clips, tape, velcro*, or self-adhesive, but few people actually know how to wrap one,

An elastic bandage provides gentle pressure on the tissue around an injury. It also gives support to the injured area, such as to protect a sprain; helps decrease pain and swelling, secure a wound bandage, or support a splint.

TIP! Wash an elastic bandage by hand and hang to dry. Do not put it in a clothes dryer.

Elastic bandage - ankle injury

Cut several horseshoe-shaped pieces of cloth or gauze for a padding around the ankle bones.(fig. 1) Hold the elastic bandage so the roll is facing up. A rolled bandage is easier to manage than a loose one.

Start with holding the loose end of the bandage on the top of the foot.(fig. 2) The first wrap should be with a mild stretch around the outside of the foot, under, and over the top so that the edge of the bandage is along the base of the toes. This first wrap will help reduce foot swelling. Always wrap the bandage in the direction of the little toe side of foot to the big toe side of the foot.(fig. 3)

Overlap the elastic bandage by one-half to one-third of its width each time you go around, and wrap the bandage moving up toward the ankle in a spiral direction, like a "figure 8". Leave the heel uncovered.

Pass the bandage around the ankle and start wrapping it in upward circles toward the knee.(fig. 4) Fasten the end to the rest of the bandage with tape, metal clips, or Velcro. Do not fasten metal clips on a bandage where there is exposed skin.

Do not wrap the bandage too tightly; it may cut off blood flow. Take off the elastic bandage at night. If you have any numbness (loss of feeling) or tingling under the elastic bandage, or if the skin becomes cold or turns blue, remove the bandage.

Hand Protection

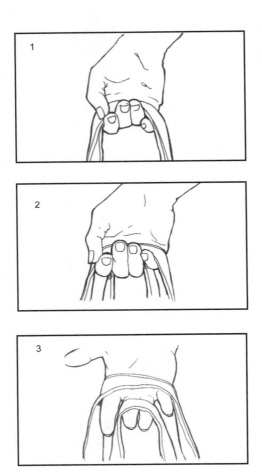

Hand Protection

In our modern times, we see more products designed to make our lives easier. One product that is now used everywhere is the plastic handled shopping bag. While it makes carrying groceries easier, it creates stressful problems for our hands. The pressure from these handles, especially when carrying heavy items, is a strain on the muscles, ligaments, bones, and tendons of the hands. This strain can cause numbness and pain in the wrist, hand and fingers. The discomfort can be compounded by conditions of arthritis and neuropathies. Here is a technique that can help reduce hand strain and discomfort.

The first picture (1) shows a typical hand position for holding a plastic bag. Notice that the weight of the bag strains the hand, and bends the fingers in an unnatural position. Now look at the second picture (2). The hand is in a normal and comfortable position. The first loop is over all four fingers, but the second loop is over only the middle and ring fingers (3). This position distributes the weight of the bag evenly over all the fingers. This technique can be used with any soft-handled bag.

The human hand and wrist have twenty-seven bones. The hands, wrists, and feet contain more than one-half the bones in the human body.

Immune System Enhancers

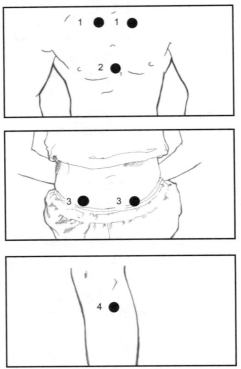

Our immune system is one of the key elements of our biochemistry that wards off infections, illness, cellular damage, and effects from stress. Protecting this important system requires regular care. Although the immune system will not deteriorate overnight. If it does deteriorate, it will require time to rebuild. Regular maintenance of this important system is the best course.

Immune System Enhancers

PRESSURE POINTS
1. Kd27 In the depression below the clavicle.

2. CV17 Center of the sternum about two
inches up from the sternum bottom.

3. B23* About three inches either side of the
spine.

4. St36* Three inches below the knee cap
and just to the outside of the shin bone.

LIFESTYLES
Manage your stress. Stress can increase from
a positive as well as a negative experience.

Trim the fat and reduce carbohydrates. Diets
high in fat can increase atherosclerosis, blood
pressure, and risk for heart disease.

Reduce salt intake. Sodium increases fluid in
the circulatory system and increases the work-
load on the heart.

AROMATHERAPY
Chamomile, lavender, lemon balm.

HELPFUL HERBS
Ginseng, **St. John's wort**, **saw palmetto.**

Heat or Cold

When an acute injury occurs, athletic trainers follow a certain procedure in order to minimize the extent and severity of the injury. A cold compress or ice is applied immediately to inhibit swelling of the inflamed tissue. After the swelling has been controlled, heat is applied to increase healing and circulation to the damaged tissue. Heat and cold are then alternated for twelve hours.

These procedures are not new. Therapists have been using them for hundreds, perhaps thousands of years. The art and science of heat and cold have been perfected in recent years, particularly in areas of sports medicine and rehabilitation.

When using a modality, such as a cold compress or ice wrap, the suggested time is up to 20 minutes. This is only a guideline and depends on individual tolerance. When using heat, moist heat is usually preferred, making the heat more effective and soothing. Care must be taken not to burn the skin when using heat.

When using either modality of heat or cold, insulating the skin is mandatory. The skin should be protected with a towel or any material that has insulating properties; cotton is best. If discomfort or swelling persists, especially with the wrist or the ankle, seek medical attention.

Heat or Cold

Studies conducted at Johns Hopkins University showed that alternating showers, when taken daily, first heat then finishing with a cold wash as could be comfortably tolerated, reduced the incidence of colds and flu after this regimen had been in place for at least thirteen weeks.

Scandinavians have been taking hot sauna baths followed by dips in chilly water for centuries. Ancient Romans, particularly soldiers, had communal bath houses where, first, one would take a hot bath heated by a nearby furnace, then finish with a cold dip, in another nearby tub, to stimulate blood circulation. The heat is said to open the pores and the cold is said to draw the blood to the surface of the skin.

Need a cold compress but do not have one handy? Go to your freezer and pull out a bag of frozen peas or small-cut vegetables. Wrap in a towel and apply to the area. The bag of vegetables conforms to the body shape and will remain cold for about 20 minutes. Monitor the area to prevent the tissue from becoming too cold. Check the area every few minutes as a precaution.

Preventing Falls.

Each year, injuries from some 170,000 falls require medical attention. Many of these falls occur with the elderly, but even toddles suffer such injuries. Here are some hints that can help prevent falls.

In the home:
Install grab bars and non-slip strips in the tub
  and shower.
Install a grab bar next to the bed for safety.
Place non-skid mats on the floor.
Install rails on stairways in and outside the
  house to keep toddlers from falling.
Provide adequate lighting and nightlights for
  hallways.
Arrange furniture for adequate space for
  walking, especially if someone is using
  a walking device.
Place gates as barriers to stairs and exits.

Out and About:
Wear appropriate footwear. Shoes with arch
  support, proper fit, and non-slip soles
  will also reduce fatigue.
Wait about one minute for eyes to adjust to
  darkened spaces, such as theaters.
Slow down. Rushing increases the fall risk.
Avoid losing balance and equilibrium. When
  standing up, wait a few seconds before
  walking. When walking, stay focused
  ahead and avoid sudden turns of the
  head or looking up.
Fatigue and over-exertion contribute to falls.

Reduce Back Pain from Lifting.

Back injuries are a major cause of lost productivity and can be a life-long aggravation. Back surgery is not always the answer to this problem. The best solution is prevention. When lifting ab object, use the following guidelines:

Make the object part of you. The closer you hold an object the more effective the body mechanics. Women who carry babies on their hip use fewer muscles less than when carrying babies in their arms.

Widen your base of support by widening the distance between your feet.

Squat, bending your knees and hips, keeping your back in correct alignment.

When lifting, use the strong muscles of your legs and not the weak muscles of your back.

Twisting as you lift can cause serious damage to your back. The spinal column and small muscles are not strong enough to withstand the pressure. Lift and turn the entire body; shift your weight to manage the object.

When lifting as a team, appoint one person to give the commands to lift, move, turn, and put down the object.

Using a support for the lower back and abdomen may help safe lifting and lessen the chance of injury.

Morning Facial Tune-up

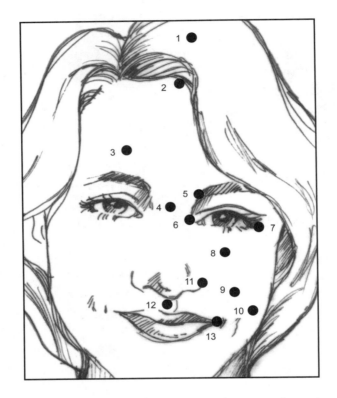

Remember that all of these points are in pairs except for the points on the Governing Vessel, GV20 (1), GV24 (2), and GV26 (12).

Morning Facial Tune-up

Here is a technique which will help you start your day on a positive note. These points will refresh and tone your skin.

Start with abdominal breathing. Twenty seconds of relaxed breathing will set the stage. I cannot over-emphasize the importance of this technique. Gently massage the following pressure points for ten seconds:

1. **GV20** Midline on top of the head.
2. **GV24** Midline at the hairline.
3. **Gb14** One inch above the center of each eye brow.
4. **Yin Tang** Bridge of the nose between the eye brows. PRESS ONLY
5. **B2** Inside corners of the eye brows. PRESS ONLY
6. **B1** Inside corner of the eye. PRESS ONLY
7. **Gb1** Outside corner of the eye. PRESS ONLY
8. **St2** One inch below the center of the eye. PRESS ONLY
9. **St7** Under the cheek bone.
10. **St6** Over the large muscle of the jaws.
11. **Li20** Groove next to the nostril. PRESS ONLY
12. **GV26** Between the nose and upper lip. PRESS ONLY
13. **St4** Corner of the mouth. PRESS ONLY

Morning Jump-start

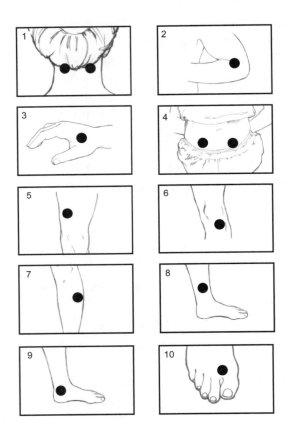

Morning Jump-start

1. **Gb20***   Wind Pool (base of the skull).
2. **LiII***   Pool at the Crook (bend of the elbow).
3. **Li4***   Adjoining Valley (web of the hand).
4. **B23***   Associated Point of Kidney (lower back).
5. **Sp10***   Sea of Blood (three inches above the knee).
6. **St36***   Three Mile Foot (three inches below knee).
7. **St40***   Abundant Splendor (beside shin bone).
8. **Sp6***   Three Yin Meeting (above ankle bone).
9. **Kd3***   Supreme Stream (behind ankle bone).
10. **Lv3***   Bigger Rushing (top of foot).

Sit in a comfortable chair. Take three or four deep breaths and relax. Begin with Gb20 and massage both points at the same time for fifteen seconds. Continue through each of the ten primary points. Li4 will have to be massaged separately. This whole exercise should take about three minutes.

When you have finished, sit back in the chair and notice that your whole body is tingling. You have wakened your neurology system with this simple massage. The morning sluggishness should be gone, and you can face your day with alertness.

Body Mass Index

The Body Mass Index is the most recent and effective measure of body weight to height. Previous calculations relied on the individual deciding whether he or she had a thin, medium, or heavy frame as a major factor in determining one's proper weight. The BMI calculates weight to height - period. You will probably need a calculator for this equation.

$$BMI = \frac{704.5 \times \text{weight in pounds}}{(\text{height in inches}) \text{ squared}}$$

For example, if you weighed 125 and were 5'2", the formula would be:

$$\frac{704.5 \times 125 \text{ or } 88062.5}{62 \times 62 \text{ or } 3844} = 22.9$$

According to your calculations, your BMI of 22.9 is Normal weight.
If you were 6 feet tall and 200 pounds, your BMI of 27.2 is Overweight.

Underweight	Under 18.5
Normal weight	18.5 to 24.9
Overweight	25 to 29.9
Obese	30 to 39.9
Severely obese	40 & over

Reduce Back Pain and Neck Strain at the Computer.

Preventing back pain and neck strain while sitting at a computer can be achieved by following a few basic rules involving proper posture of the head, forearms, back, and feet:
The first step is to adjust the chair to an appropriate height.
The head should be level with the monitor and the top of the screen at eye level.
The forearms should be parallel to the keyboard and held slightly above it.
The lower back should be supported by a small pillow or folded towel between the back of the chair and the lower back.
Feet should rest flat on the floor or footrest.
Arrange computer desk and equipment so as to reduce glare from windows and overhead lights.
Set the monitor about 24 inches away from the person.

If you share a computer station with someone else, make all the necessary adjustments before you start working. This will reduce pain, discomfort, tension, and strain. Work will be more efficient and less fatiguing.

Neck Roll

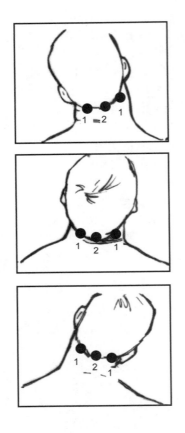

Neck Roll

PRESSURE POINTS
1. **Gb20*** At the base of the skull one inch
   either side of the spine.

2. **GV16** Midline at the base of the skull.

Many of the headaches that we experience
are caused by neck problems; the cervical
spine is misaligned or neck muscles are tense
or sore from over-exertion. The neck and
cervical spine is a complex network of nerves,
vessels, intricate muscles, and soft tissue. The
highest concentration of red muscle fibers are
in the hands, feet and neck. Red muscle fibers
are the muscle fibers that control strength,
coordination and endurance. Those areas of
the body that have the highest concentration
are centers for skilled activities. When they
become over-exerted, they can cause pain
and discomfort.
   In addition to the acupressure points of
the back of the neck, performing a few simple
head rolls can increase circulation, stretch and
energize tired muscles, and help to realign the
cervical vertebrae. Tilt your head back as if
you were looking at the ceiling. Gently roll
your head from side to side, gently massaging
pressure points Gb20* and GV16. Do this
head roll several times for a quick stress
reducer.

Quick Tip for Tired Eyes

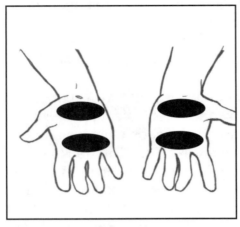

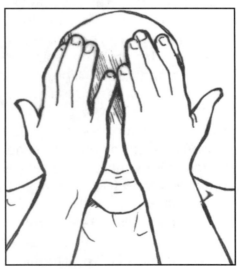

Quick Tip for Tired Eyes

Only have ten seconds to refresh? Try this quick massage to rejuvenate your eyes and help in focusing. Place both palms over your eyes without the palms touching the eyelids. With mild to moderate pressure move the hands in small circles massaging above and below the eyes. Move one hand in a clockwise direction and the other hand counterclockwise.

Try not to pinch the nose during this motion. During this massage you will be stimulating eight pressure points. If you have a few extra seconds, press Yin Tang, the bridge of the nose between the eyebrows.

Shutting your eyes for a few minutes or even several seconds will refocus them and ease the strain. Blinking soothes and moistens the eyes and eases tight eye muscles. Certain over-the-counter eye products are actually decongestant and can further dry your eyes, so avoid them.

For tired eyes, wash them with cold water several times a day. This treatment reduces inflammation, relaxes the eyes, and provides relief from eyestrain and fatigue.

Lavender oil gently relieves tired and strained eyes. Fill a container with two cups of warm water and add one drop of lavender oil. Soak two cotton pads in the mixed solution, squeeze out excess water, and place one pad over each closed eye for ten minutes.

Rejuvenate Tired Hands

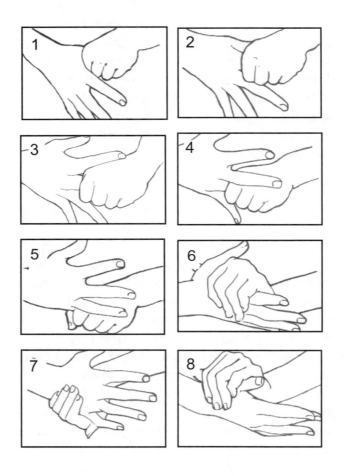

Rejuvenate Tired Hands

These are quick and easy exercises that can re-energize your hands when they are tired from physical activity or repetitive movements. These exercises increase circulation and reduce hand stress. Follow the picture sequence and do not forget to remove rings before these exercises.

Start with the thumb and hold each hand position for five seconds using a squeezing motion. Then begin at the finger tip and massage the fingers of the other hand in a pulsating motion to the base of each finger. Massaging from the tip to the base of each finger stimulates circulation and reduces swelling. This can sometimes be easier using a light oil or hand cream.

The palms of the hands contain many small muscles called *intrinsic muscles.* These muscles perform sophisticated movements and can fatigue from overuse. Hands become stiff and sore and joints experience pain from over-exertion. Figures 6, 7, and 8 illustrate how to massage the palms to rejuvenate these   muscles and joints and to relieve pain and fatigue.

Suggested Readings

Acupressure Techniques by Julian Kenyan, MD. 1994 Healing Arts Press. Rochester, Vermont.

Acupressure's Potent Points by Michael Reed Gach, PhD. 1990 Bantam Book. New York.

A Complete Guide to Acupressure by Iona Marsaa Teeyuarden, MA. 1996 Japan Publications, Inc. Tokyo.

Fundamentals of Therapeutic Massage by Sandy Fritz. 1999 Mosby-Year Book. St. Louis, Missouri.

Hands-On Healing by Lewis Harrison. 1998 Kensington Publishing Corporation. New York.

Healing with Pressure Point Therapy by Steve Shimer, L Ac. 1999 Prentice Hall Publishing Company. Paramus, New Jersey.

The New Healing Herbs by Michael Castleman. 2001 Rodale, Inc. Emmaus, PA.

Prescription for Herbal Healing by Phyllis A. Balch, CNC. 2002 Avery, a member of Penguin Putnam, Inc. New York.

References

Akamasu, E. 1970. Modern Oriental Drugs. Yishiyakusha, Tokyo, Japan

Artiges, A. 1991. What are the legal requirements for the use of phytopharmaceutical drugs in France? J. Ethnopharmacol. 32:231-234.

Arvigo, R., and M. Balick. 1993. Rainforest Remedies: 100 Healing Herbs of Belize. Lotus Press, Twin Lakes, WI

Beckstrom-Sternberg, S.M., and J.A. Duke. 1994. Potential for synergistic action of phytochemicals in spices. In G. Charalambous, ed. Spices, Herbs, and Edible Fungi. Elsevier Sciences B.V., New York, NY

Bensky, D. and A. Gamble. 1993. Chinese Herbal Medicine: Materia Medica (revised edition). Eastland Press Inc., Seattle, WA

Blumenthal, Mark 2005
ABC Clinical Guide to Herbs, American Botanical Council,, Austin, TX

References

Bode, J.C., U. Schmidt, and H.K. Durr. 1977. Silymarin for the treatment of acute viral hepatitis Med. Klin. 72:513-518.

Braunig, B., M. Dorn, Limburg, E. Knick, and Bausendorf. 1992. Echinacea purpureae radix for strengthening the immune response in flu-like infections. Zeitschrift fhr Phytotherapie 13:7-13.

Buchman, D.D. 1980. Herbal Medicine. Gramercy Publishing Company, New York, NY

Catlin, D.H., M. Sekera, and D.C. Adelman. 1993. Erythroderma associated with the ingestion of an herbal product. West. J. Med. 159:491-493.

Champpault, G., J.D. Patel, and A.M. Bonnard. 1984. A double-blind trial of an extract of the plant Serenoo repens in benign prostatic hyperplasia. Br. J. Clin. Pharmacol. 18(3):461-462.

Chaudhury, R.R. 1992. Herbal Medicine for Human Health. World Health Organization (SEARO, No. 20).

References

Chopra, R.N., and I.C. Chopra. 1959. A review of work on Indian medicinal plants. Indian Council of Medical Research Special Report Series No. 1, pp. 99, 107.

Corsi, S. 1987. Report on Trial of Bilberry Anthocyanosides (Tegens-inverni della beffa) in the Medical Treatment of Venous Insufficiency of the Lower Limbs. Casa di Cura S. Chiara, Florence, Italy.

Dahanukar, S.A., S.M. Karandikar, and M. Desai. 1984. Efficacy of Piper longum in childhood asthma. Indian Drugs 21:384-388.

Duke, J.A. 1986. Handbook of Northeastern Indian Medicinal Plants. Quarterman Press, Lincoln, MA.

Duke, J.A. 1988. Handbook of Nuts. CRC Press, Inc., Boca Raton, FL.

Duke, J.A. 1989. Ginseng: A Concise Handbook. Reference Publications Inc., Algonac, MI.

Duke, J.A. 1992a. Handbook of Phytochemical Constituents of GRAS Herbs and Other Economic Plants. CRC Press, Inc., Boca Raton, FL.

References

Duke, J.A. 1992b. Handbook of Biologically
Active Phytochemicals and Their Activities.
CRC Press, Inc., Boca Raton, FL.

Duke, J.A., and R.V. Martinez. In press.
Amazonian ethnobotanical dictionary. In
Handbook of Ethnobotanicals (Peru). CRC
Press, Inc., Boca Raton, FL.

Farnsworth, N.R., O. Akerele, A.S. Bingel,
D.D. Soejarta, and Z. Eno. 1985. Medicinal
plants in therapy. Bull. World Health Organ.
63(6):965-981.

Farnsworth, N.R., and R.W. Morris. 1976.
Higher plants: the sleeping giant of drug
development. Am. J. Pharm. March/April:46.

Feher, H., et al. 1990. Hepaprotective activity
of   silymarin therapy in patients with chronic alcoholic liver disease. Orv. Hetil. 130:51.

Gilhooley, M. 1989. Pharmaceutical drug
regulation in China. Food Drug Cosmetic Law
Journal 44:21-39.

Haas, H. 1981. Brain disorders and vasoactive
substances of plant origin. Planta Medical.
(Suppl.):257-265.

References

Han, B.H., M.H. Park, L.K. Woo, W.S. Woo, and Y.N. Han. 1979. Studies on antioxidant components of Korean ginseng. Korean Biochemistry Journal 12(1):33
.

Handbook of Domestic Medicine and Common Ayurvedic Remedies. 1979. Central Council for Research in Indian Medicine and Homeopathy, New Delhi, India. pp. 91-112.

Hirayama, T. 1986. Nutrition and cancer--a large scale cohort study. Prog. Clin. Biol. Res. 206:299-311.

Kao, F.F. 1992. The impact of Chinese medicine on America. Am. J. Chin. Med. 20(1):1-16.

Kirkland, J., H.F. Mathews, C.W. Sullivan III, and K. Baldwin, eds. 1992. Herbal and Magic Medicine: Traditional Healing Today. Duke University Press, Durham, N.C., and London.

Kulkarni, R.R., P.S. Patki, V.P. Jog, S.G. Gandage, and B. Patwardhan. 1991. Treatment of osteoarthritis with a herbomineral formulation: a double-blind, placebo-controlled, cross-over study. J. Ethnopharmacol. 33:91-95.

References

Liu, C., and P. Xiao. 1992. Recent advances on ginseng research in China. J. Ethnopharmacol. 36:27-38.

Majno, G.M. 1975. Healing Hand: Man and Wound in the Ancient World. Harvard University Press, Cambridge, MA.

Moerman, D.C. 1982. Geraniums for the Iroquois. A Field Guide to American Indian Medicinal Plants. Reference Publications, Algonac, MI, 242 pp.

Money Magazine, Special Edition, 2003, Time Life Publicatins, New York, NY.

Mousavi, Y., and H. Adlercreutz. 1993. Genistein is an effective stimulator of sex hormone-binding globulin production in hepatocarcinoma human liver cancer cells and suppresses proliferation of these cells in culture. Steroids 58:301-304.

Perry, L.M. 1980. Medicinal Plants of East and Southeast Asia: Attributed Properties and Uses. MIT Press, Cambridge, MA.

References

Raabe, A., M. Raabe, and P. Ihm. 1991. Therapeutic follow-up using automatic per-imery in chronic cerebroretinal ischemia in eld-erly tpatients: prospective double-blind study with graduated dose Ginkgo biloba treatment (EGb 761). Klin. Monatsbl. Augenheilkd. 199(6):432-438.

Rai, G.S., C. Shovlin, and K.A. Wesnes. 1991. A double-blind, placebo-controlled study of Ginkgo   biloba extract in elderly outpatients with mild to   moderate memory impair-ment. Curr. Med. Res. Opin. 12(6):350-355.

Schaffler, K., and P. Reeh. 1985. Long-term drug administration effects of Ginkgo biloba on the
performance of healthy subjects exposed to hypoxia. In Effects of Ginkgo Biloba Extracts on Organic Cerebral Impairment. Eurotext Ltd., London.

Snider, S. 1991. Beware the unknown brew: herbal teas and toxicity. FDA Consumer (May):31-33.

Starfield, Barbara, MD, MPH, Department of Health Policy and Management, Johns Hopkins School of Hygiene and Public Health JAMA, July, 2000. 284:483-485.

References

Sumathikutty, M.A., K. Rajaraman, B. Sankarikutty, and A.G. Mathew. 1979. Chemical composition of pepper grades and products. Journal of Food Science and Technology 16:249-254.

Swanston-Flatt, S.K., C. Day, P.R. Flott, et al. 1989. Glycemic effects of traditional European plant treatments for diabetes: studies in normal and streptozotocin diabetic mice. Diabetes Res. 10(2):69-73.

Taillandier, J. 1988. Ginkgo biloba extract in the treatment of cerebral disorders due to aging. In E.W. Funfgeld, ed. Rokan (Ginkgo Biloba): Recent Results in Pharmacology and Clinic. Springer-Verlag, Berlin.

Tsumura, A. 1991. Kampo, How the Japanese Updated Traditional Herbal Medicine. Japan Publications, Inc., Tokyo and New York.

Ura, H., T. Obara, K. Okamura, and M. Namiki. 1993. Growth inhibition of pancreatic cancer cells by flavonoids. Gan To Kagaku Ryoho 20(13):2083-2085.

Vogel, V.L. 1970. American Indian Medicine. University of Oklahoma Press, Norman, OK.

References

Wall Street Journal. 1993. Vital statistics: disputed cost of creating a drug. November 9.

Wang, B.X., J.C. Cui, and A.J. Lui. 1980. The effect of polysaccharides of root of Panax ginseng on the immune function. Acta Pharmaceutica Sinica 17:312-320.

Weitbrecht, W.V., and W. Jansen. 1985. Doubleblind and comparative (Ginkgo biloba versus placebo) therapeutic study in geriatric patients with primary degenerative dementia-- a preliminary evaluation. In A. Agnoli et al., eds. Effects of Ginkgo Biloba Extract on Organic Cerebral Impairment. John Libbey Eurotext Ltd., London.

Witte, S., I. Anadere, and E. Walitza. 1992. Improvement of hemorheology with Ginkgo biloba extract: decreasing a cardiovascular risk factor. Fortschr. Med. 110(13):247-250.

World Health Organization. 1991. Guidelines for the Assessment of Herbal Medicines. Programme on Traditional Medicines, Geneva.

World POPClock from US Bureau of the Census U.S. Census Bureau, Population DivisionMaintained By: Information & Research Services

References

Yanagihara, K., A. Ito, T. Toge, and M. Numoto. 1993. Antiproliferative effects of isoflavones on human cancer cell lines established from the gastrointestinal tract. Cancer Res. 53(23):5815-5821.

Youngken, H.W. 1950. A Textbook of Pharmacognosy. McGraw-Hill, New York.

Zhang, J.T. 1989. Progress of research on three kinds of anti-aging drugs. Information of the Chinese
Pharmacological Society 6(3-4):4.

Index

Index

Index

Index

Index

Index

Index

Appendix A
Aromatherapy -
Essences & Oils

The following is the list of the symptoms mentioned in Section Two and the essential oils and herbs that are recommended for treatment.

Allergies   chamomile

Angina   hawthorn berry, ginger

Anxiety   orange blossom,
                         tangerine

Arthritis   juniper, eucalyptus

Asthma   eucalyptus, coffee

Back pain   sandalwood

Bad breath   peppermint

Constipation   lavender, geranium

Cough, colds   sage

Depression   orange blossom,
                         lemon balm

Aromatherapy - Essences & Oils

Diarrhea	geranium
Dizziness	peppermint
Earache	lavender
Eye strain	apply a cold compress with a solution of linden blossom
Fatigue	peppermint
Fever	lavender
Headache	orange blossom, lemon balm
Hemorrhoids	chamomile
Hiccups	clove
High blood pressure	orange blossom
Indigestion	peppermint
Insomnia	lavender, rosemary
Joint pain	juniper, eucalyptus

Aromatherapy -
Essences & Oils

Leg cramps   rosemary

Low blood
     pressure   rosemary

Menstrual cramps   rosemary, lavender

Migraines   marjoram

Nausea,
  motion sickness   ginger, peppermint

Neck/Shoulder
     tension   lavender, chamomile

Pain   chamomile, licorice

Sinusitis   eucalyptus, chamomile

Sore throat   sandalwood

Stress   lavender,
                      orange blossom

Tennis elbow   chamomile

Toothache   clove

Aromatherapy -
Essences & Oils

CAUTION!
Using aromatherapy during the first trimester
of pregnancy may be harmful. Consult your
healthcare professional.

CAUTION!
Essential oils should not be taken internally
without the guidance of a physician or
licensed practitioner.

Studies have shown that <u>Lavender</u> has a
positive effect on women to stimulate sexual
interest. Men seem to respond in kind to the
aroma of <u>Cinnamon</u>.

Appendix B
Anatomical References of the Human Body.

The following pages contain some references to the anatomical orientation of the human body. The anatomical orientations are commonly used when studying anatomy and physiology. The Western anatomical position depicts the human body standing upright and arms at the sides with palms of the hands facing forward. This anatomical position is more commonly seen in the Western cultures, and is the one selected for teaching, studying, examining. and describing the human anatomy.

      The Eastern anatomical position depicts the human body upright with arms raised over the head and palms of the hands facing forward. This is an important disctinction for understanding and using the meridians of the human body. Knowing this anatomical orientations of the human body is helpful understanding the Eastern philosophy of using acupressure and acupuncture. When the arms are raised over the head, the Yin and Yang meridians and pressure points numbers flow in the correct directions. The Western standard of the anatomical position is most commonly used in the United States, but the Eastern version is used when studying and applying acupressure.

Anatomical References of the Human Body

The anatomical position of the human body is a standardized description of the human body. In Western cultures. This position is usually illustrated with the body upright and arms at the sides with the palms of the hands facing forward. The human body is divided by three planes for standard reference. The *frontal plane* divides the body side to side. The *coronal plane* divides the body front to back, and the *saggital plane* divides the body top to bottom. These three planes divide the body so that any point in or on the body can be exactly located for examining or referencing.

In some Eastern cultures, the anatomical position of the human body is displayed with the body upright and the arms raised over the head with palms facing forward. This is a variation from the Western anatomical position, but it is an important distinction. Visualizing the arms raised over the head positions all the meridians of the arms and their pressure points in correct directions. The Yin and Yang meridians flow in the up and down direction and the pressure point numbers are in sequence. When viewing the six meridians of the upper extremities with arms over the head, the descending and ascending numbers of the pressure points are also easier to locate on the body.

Anatomical References of the Human Body

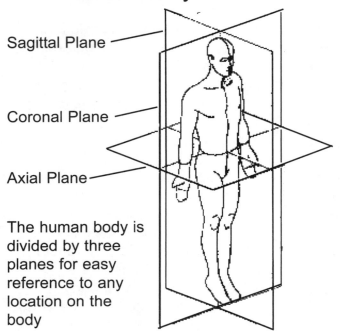

Sagittal Plane

Coronal Plane

Axial Plane

The human body is divided by three planes for easy reference to any location on the body

Sagittal Plane (Lateral Plane) A verticle plane running from front to back; divides the body into right and left sides.

Coronal Plane (Frontal Plane) A verticle plane running from side to side; divides the body into anterior and posterior portions.

Axial Plane (Transverse Plane) A horizontal plane; divides the body into upper and lower parts.

Anatomical References of the Human Body

Directional terms describe the positions of structures relative to other structures or locations in the body.

Superior or cranial
toward the head end of the body or upper (for example, the hand is part of the superior extremity)

Inferior or caudal
away from the head or lower (for example, the foot is part of the inferior extremity)

Anterior or ventral
front (for example, the kneecap is located on the anterior side of the leg)

Posterior or dorsal
back (for example, the shoulder blades are located on the posterior side of the body)

Medial
toward the midline of the body (for example, the great toe is located at the medial side of the foot)

Lateral
away from the midline of the body (for example, the little toe is located at the lateral side of the foot)

Appendix C
Definition of Terms

Cold compress
In preparing a cold compress, fill a bowl
with cold water, 45-50 degrees F.
Add a few drops of essential oil to the water,
such as lavender or lemon
balm. (optional)
Dip a folded piece of clean cotton cloth into
the prepared water.
Squeeze out excess water.
Place the moistened cloth onto the affected
area until it reaches body temperature.
Cold compresses are helpful for headaches,
neck tension, sprains, and strains.

Hot compress
In preparing a hot compress, fill a bowl
with hot water, 95-100 degrees F.
Add a few drops of essential oil, such as
lavender or lemon balm. (optional)
Dip a folded piece of clean cotton cloth into
the prepared water.
Squeeze out excess water.
Place the moistened cloth onto the affected
area until it reaches room temperature.
Compresses at body temperature, 98.6
degrees F. will feel warm on the skin.
Hot water above 100 degrees F. can
cause damage to sensitive, such as
ears, eyes and genital areas.

Definition of Terms

Essences

Condensed flavors are made as their flowers, buds, leaves, or fruit are distilled or pressed, then mixed with water or alcohol. Examples are almond extract, lemon extract, and rose water.

Infusion

A liquid produced by soaking herbs in hot, not boiling, water, such as a tea, brew, or potion.

Tea made by steeping an herb's leaves or flowers in hot water.

Moist heat

Moist heat is a hot compress with water that, when applied to the skin, provides deep heat to muscles and tissue for relief from aches and pain.

Dry heat, such as a heating pad or hot water bottle, is without moisture. Dry heat is a gentler heat that slowly penetrates the body and used for stomach aches, nausea, or as a warmer on a cold night.

Poultice

A soft, moist mass applied to the skin to provide heat and moisture.

An herbal paste spread on a cloth and applied externally to the body.

Definition of Terms

Oils & oil extracts

Oil extracts are made from fresh herbs that
    contain volatile oils used for healing.
Fresh herbs are necessary for extracting the
    oils and are usually crushed with a
    mortar and pestle. Olive or sesame oil
    is then added, at the rate of one pint
    of oil to every two ounces of herbs. The
    mixture is allowed to stand in a warm
    place, out of direct light, for three days.
    The oils are stored in dark, air-tight,
    glass containers.
Add one to two capsules of Vitamin E to each
    bottle for preserving the extracted oils.

Tincture

An herb extract steeped in alcohol for several
    weeks, and available commercially and
    usually taken in drops.
An alcoholic solution of a medicinal substance.
A water and alcohol concentration of a plant
    used either for convenience, or
    because some active ingredients
    are not very soluble in a tea.